# Lactogenic immunity in the sow

## A PRACTICAL APPROACH

For this English edition:
Lactogenic immunity in the sow. A practical approach

Plaza Antonio Beltrán Martínez nº 1, planta 8 - letra I
(Centro empresarial El Trovador)
50002 Zaragoza - Spain

First printing: March 2018

This book has been published originally in Spanish under the title:
*Inmunidad lactogénica en la cerda. Enfoque práctico*
© 2018 Grupo Asís Biomedia, S.L.
ISBN Spanish edition: 978-84-17225-28-5

Translation:
Chef du Monde

Illustrator:
Jacob Gragera Artal

ISBN: 978-84-17225-43-8
D.L.: Z 335-2018

Design, layout and printing:
Servet editorial - Grupo Asís Biomedia, S.L.
www.grupoasis.com
info@grupoasis.com

GRUPO asis

**Servet is the publishing house of Grupo Asís**



Warning:

Veterinary science is constantly evolving, as are pharmacology and the other sciences. Inevitably, it is therefore the responsibility of the veterinary surgeon to determine and verify the dosage, the method of administration, the duration of treatment and any possible contraindications to the treatments given to each individual patient, based on his or her professional experience. Neither the publisher nor the author can be held liable for any damage or harm caused to people, animals or properties resulting from the correct or incorrect application of the information contained in this book.

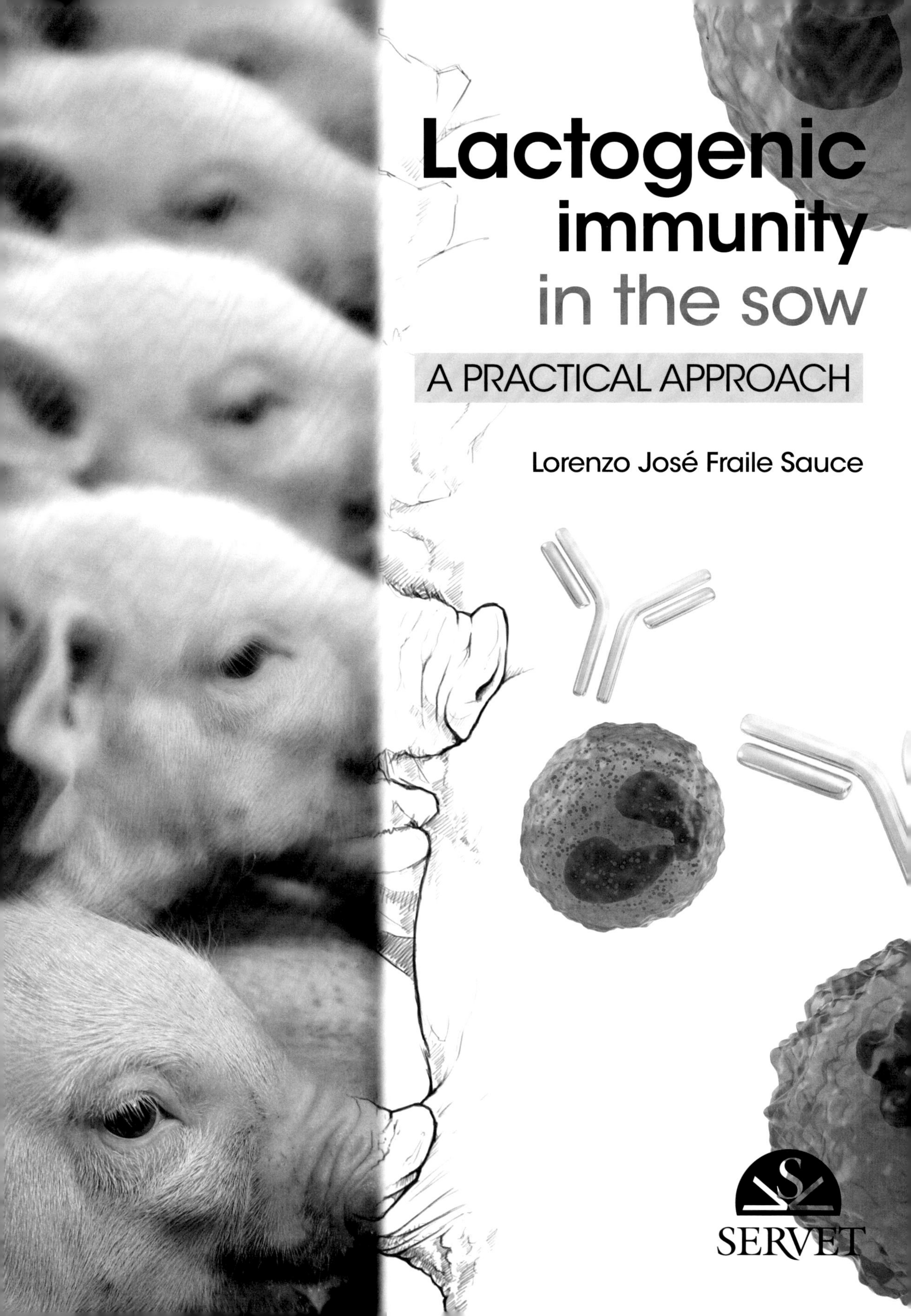

# Lactogenic immunity in the sow

## A PRACTICAL APPROACH

Lorenzo José Fraile Sauce

SERVET

*This book is dedicated to my family, Pily, Pablo and Teresa,*
*whose sacrifices and love have made it all possible.*

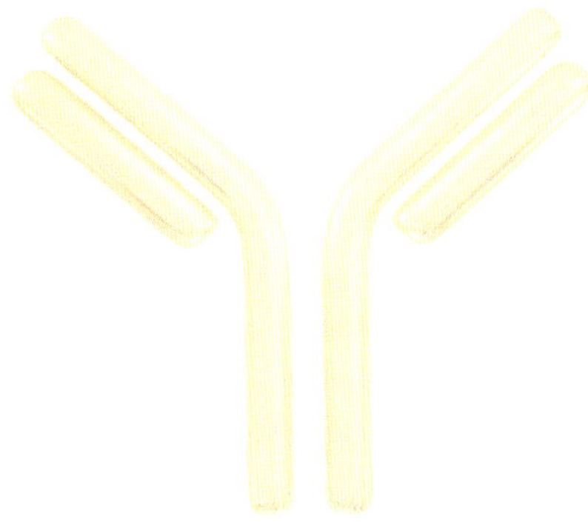

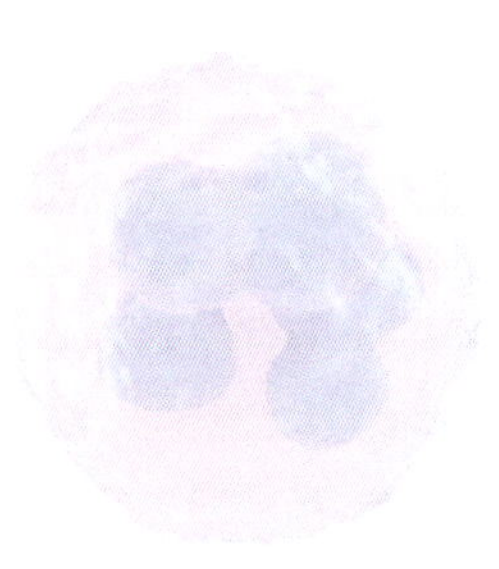

# ACKNOWLEDGEMENTS

I would like to thank everyone:

- Who have provided the daily stability and support I needed to carry out my work. I would particularly like to thank my wife, Pily, and my children, Pablo and Teresa, for their endless love, enormous understanding and patience with me.
- Those who have helped me acquire the immunological knowledge required to write this book. I would like to make special mention of María Montoya, one of the best immunologists I have ever met.
- Those who have helped me gain such a wealth of experience of on–farm preventative medicine programmes in pigs. I would particularly like to thank Don Santiago Bernaus i Gaset for giving me the opportunity to work for his company (Picber S.A.), and for the confidence he has always placed in me.
- All those who have helped me complete this project. I would like to thank all the editorial team at Servet.

Thank you all so much.

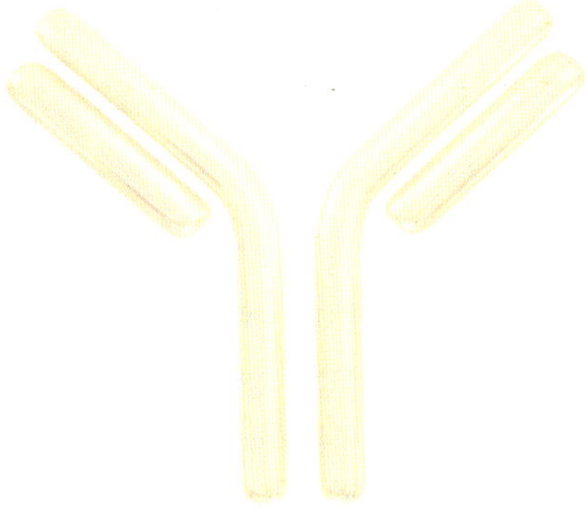

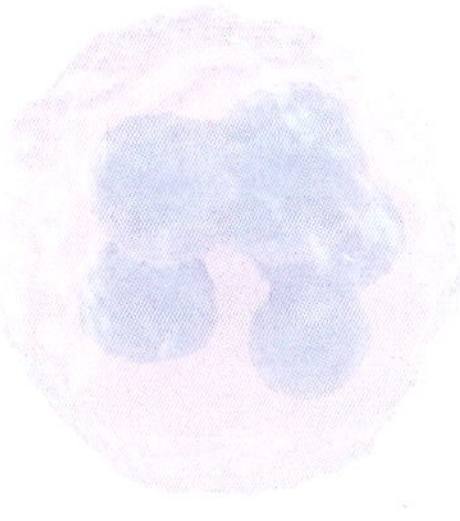
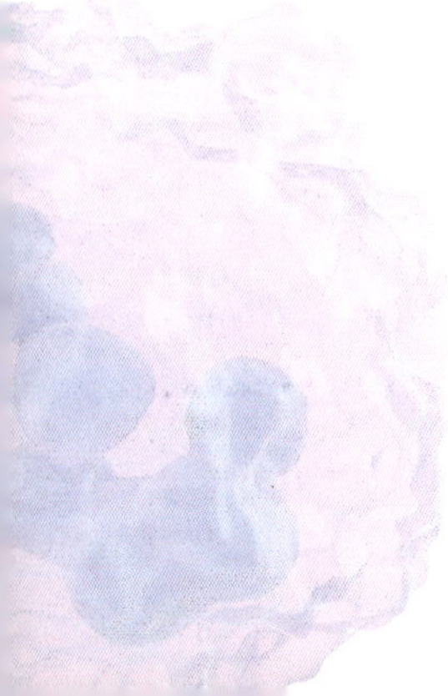

# THE AUTHOR

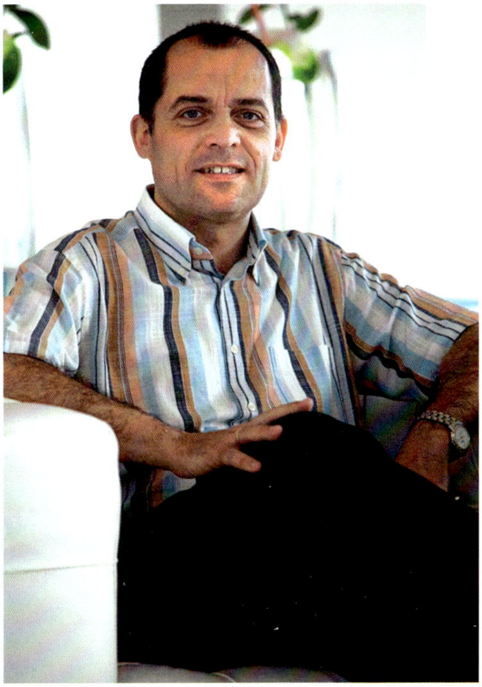

## LORENZO JOSÉ FRAILE SAUCE

Degree in Veterinary Medicine (1992) and Doctor of Veterinary Pharmacology in 1996, both from the University of Zaragoza, Spain, then specialist pig vet for Cargill España S.A. and Picber S.A. until 2004.

Researcher at the *Centre de Recerca en Sanitat Animal* (CReSA; Centre for Animal Health Research) from 2004 to 2010, where he was head of the Department of Epidemiology, Disease Control and Clinical Trials. Collaborator with the European Medicines Agency from 2005 to 2007, assessing veterinary medicines submitted for registration in Europe through his work on the Committee for Medicinal Products for Veterinary Use (CVMP). Member of the Scientific Advice Group on Antimicrobials, which provides scientific advice on all aspects of the use of antimicrobials in veterinary medicine to CVMP, from 2006 to 2007.

Adjunct professor of Epidemiology and Pharmacology at the University of Lleida since 2010, and involved in teaching the Masters Degree in Swine Production and Health offered by the Complutense University of Madrid, the University of Lleida and the University of Zaragoza. His current fields of scientific interest are epidemiology, immunology and clinical pharmacology, and his research aims to optimise preventative medicine programmes in pigs. He is the author of over 80 articles published in international scientific journals and 130 papers presented at national and international conferences. Finally, he has been a speaker at many veterinary conventions.

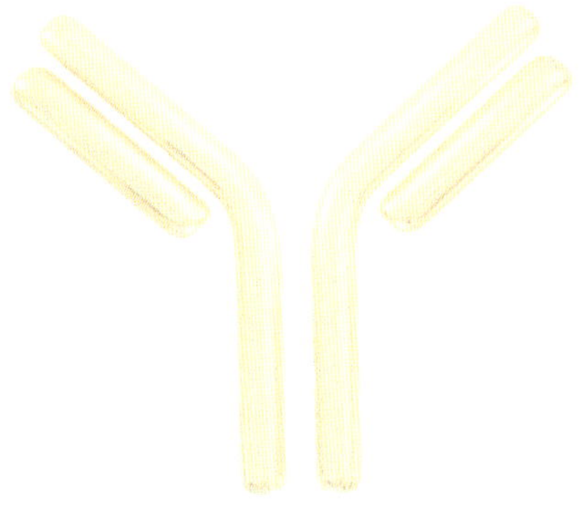

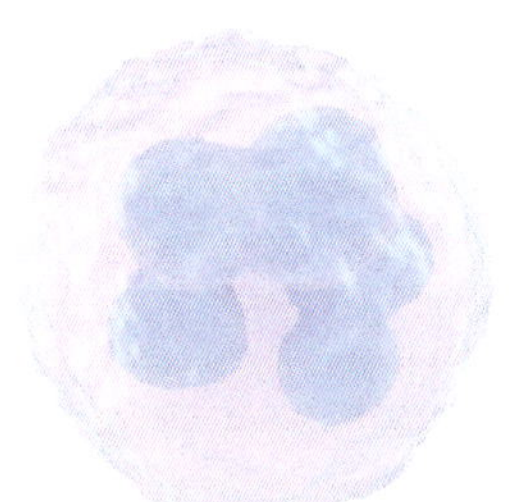

# FOREWORD

Genetic improvement in areas such as more prolific litters has generated various processes to adapt to the changing situation in pig production in recent years. The milk–producing ability of the sow has not increased in line with the number of piglets born. But it remains true that the individual intake of colostrum and milk is the main factor limiting piglet immunisation through the colostrum.

Colostrum is important as a source of immunoglobulins that help the piglet overcome the challenges presented by contact with pathogens in the weeks after birth. Given this, it is essential to understand the mechanisms that determine the quantity and quality of the colostrum, and following this, the milk produced. The objective is for the piglet to be properly immunised through its mother's milk. This will help as part of any pig disease control programme and must complement a sow vaccination programme. Piglet vaccination can then be tailored, taking into account this period of acquired maternal immunity.

Many factors affect the process of lactogenic (milk–derived) immunity, including mechanisms that start weeks before birth. This book covers all of the issues that affect this process, including nutritional, metabolic and disease factors.

Lorenzo Fraile has a wealth of expertise and has published many articles on veterinary medicine and pharmacology. He also has considerable practical experience of managing processes and conditions on farm. This book provides the reader with a guide to help them tackle the challenges that arise in their daily work much more effectively.

It is my sincere desire and conviction that this book will enlighten all those that read it.

**Jordi Baliellas Capdevila**
Veterinary surgeon

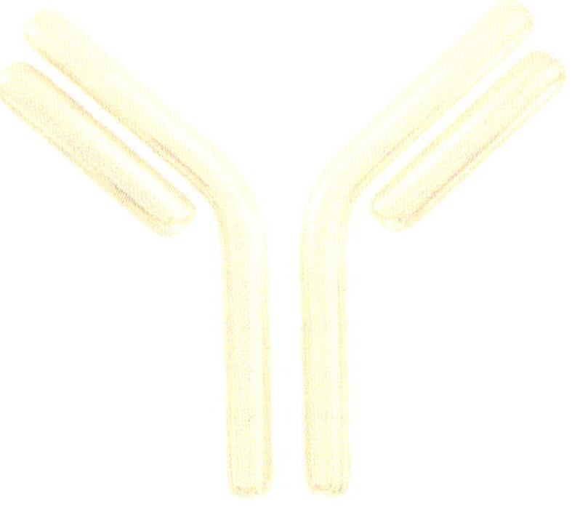

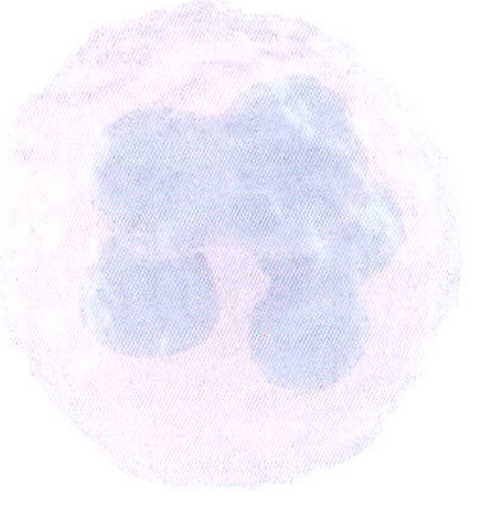

# PREFACE

I have been a practising veterinary surgeon for many years and I have always intended to write something that would combine my clinical experience using vaccines with theoretical knowledge about immunology. I have always believed that science and clinical practice should complement one another. The scientist should be familiar with clinical practice in order to design their research projects, and the veterinary clinician should never forget the science underpinning their profession. The control of many pig diseases is currently based on vaccinating the sow and transmitting this immunity to the piglet. Therefore, it is very important that the clinician should have a complete understanding of the immunological mechanisms on which this strategy of preventative medicine is based.

In this book on lactogenic immunity in sows, I have attempted to present a simple, up–to–date and practical approach to the most important factors that a practising veterinary surgeon should take into account when designing effective preventative medicine programmes in pigs. So basic, practical immunological concepts are evaluated and pig disease control programmes based on vaccination of both the sow and the piglet are discussed. I wrote this book with my veterinary colleagues in mind; it is dedicated to clinical practice, in the hope that it will be a useful tool for consultation. I will count it a success if it prompts the veterinary clinician to reflect on the whys and wherefores of the vaccines they are administering, and question themselves on how they employ these vaccines in order to optimise their everyday use.

**Lorenzo José Fraile Sauce**

# TABLE OF CONTENTS



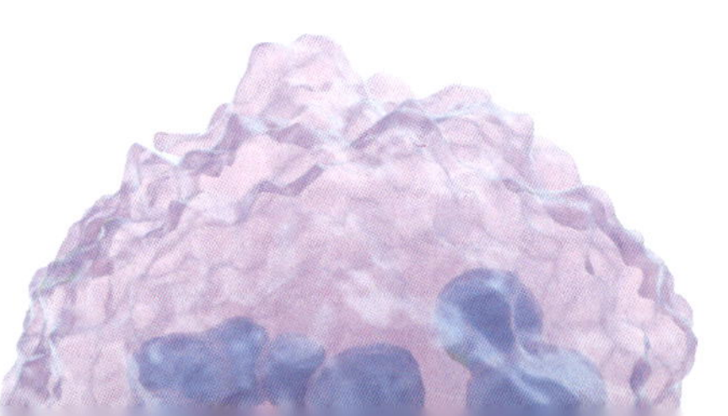

## 03 TRANSFER OF PASSIVE IMMUNITY TO THE PIGLET 43

# 04 PREVENTION PROGRAMMES IN PIGS 73



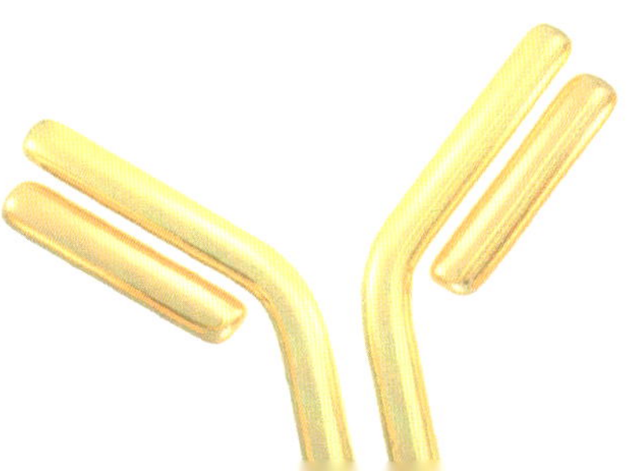

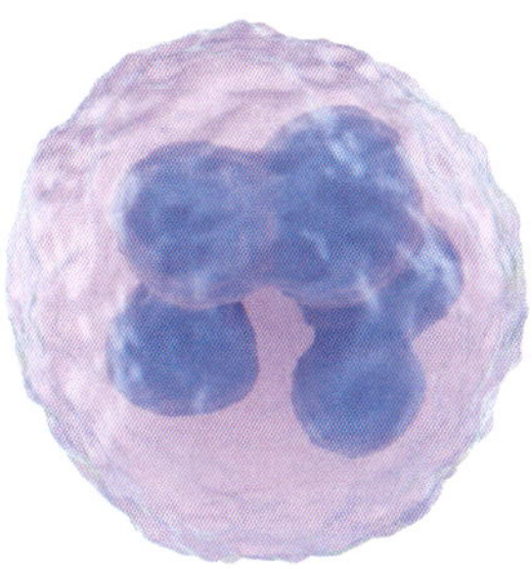

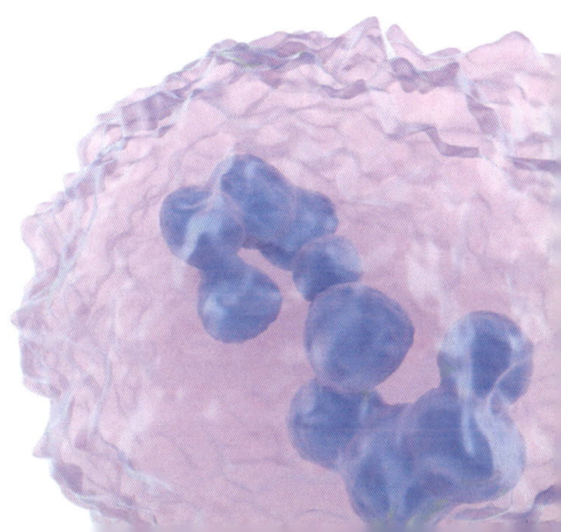

# 01

# INTRODUCTION

# INTRODUCTION

## BASIC IMMUNOLOGICAL CONCEPTS

Immunology as we know it is a relatively new science. Its origin is attributed to the English doctor, Edward Jenner, in the eighteenth century. In the year 1796, with smallpox at its height right across Europe, Edward Jenner noticed that milkmaids occasionally acquired a kind of 'cowpox' through continuous contact with their cows, and that they were subsequently protected against smallpox. Jenner took a sample of 'cowpox' from the hand of one of these milkmaids, and injected the fluid into the hand of an 8-year-old boy, James Phipps. After Phipps had recovered from a very mild illness 48 days later, Jenner injected him with human smallpox, but this time the boy showed no sign of the disease. Jenner called this process vaccination. This methodology, which would of course be unacceptable from an ethical perspective today, helped demonstrate the great potential of vaccination to control infectious diseases. Later, Louis Pasteur (1822–1895) studied Jenner's work and started to inject attenuated microorganisms into animals. In 1881, 5 years after *Bacillus anthracis* was described by Robert Koch (1843–1910), Pasteur conducted a simple experiment in Pouilly-le-Fort. Highly virulent preparations of the anthrax bacillus were injected into 48 sheep and 10 cows, after prior vaccination of 24 of the sheep and 6 of the cows with inactivated preparations of the same bacteria. All of the vaccinated animals resisted the disease, while all of the unvaccinated animals died. Thus, the anthrax vaccine was invented. The news found its way around the world, and Pasteur started on a brilliant career that would culminate in products that included vaccines for fowl cholera and rabies. Pasteur introduced the terms 'vaccine' and 'vaccination' that are still used today to describe the inoculation of healthy individuals with strains of infectious agents that have been attenuated or modified to generate protection against that disease. At the start of the twentieth century, the existence of 'immunity' to infectious agents was a recognised fact, and ever since then, the science that has identified many of the immune system's molecular and cellular mechanisms has continued to develop.

The immune system's main objective is to differentiate between the animal's own body and foreign material, so it has to establish mechanisms to constantly check and recognise all the biomolecular structures within any type of organism. Once a foreign structure is detected, one or more responses to this structure are triggered.

Immunology is the study of the mechanisms used by the body to defend itself against infectious agents and other foreign substances in the environment.

There is a wide range of invasive microorganisms, including bacteria, viruses, fungi, protozoa and helminths. Many of these microorganisms, when they come across an ideal niche where they can survive in the animal's body, try to colonise it. Some have developed a range of strategies to do this, but invasive infectious agents can only survive and succeed if they manage to evade the immune system of the colonised animal (the host) long enough to reproduce and transmit their progeny to a new host. The host must control and/or remove the invasive agent which is under great selective pressure: either it finds a host, or it dies. Survival of an animal depends on the defensive barriers that it uses against invasive microorganisms, and organisms that do not manage to evade the immune system will not survive and will be removed. These defensive measures are essential for survival, so a wide range of mechanisms have evolved to ensure an effective response. Some of these functions have evolved against multiple invasive microorganisms, while others are specific to just a few. Some work at the surface of the body to prevent entry, and others work inside the body to destroy any pathogenic microorganisms that manage to overcome the defensive barriers on the surface. Some mechanisms work against invading bacteria, some against viruses that live within the host's cells, and others have been developed against larger invaders, such as fungi, helminths and insects.

It is important to emphasise that only a small proportion of organisms cause disease in animals, and these are called pathogens. Pathogens vary greatly in their virulence, and have an ability to introduce disease with varying degrees of severity. A highly virulent organism is one that can evade or overcome the immune system more effectively and cause a more serious disease than a mildly virulent organism. Mildly virulent pathogens only cause disease if they are administered in very high concentrations, or if the immune system is compromised for some reason.

In general, the immune system has various modes of defensive barrier, such as the skin, protective chemicals in the blood and body fluids, and physiological reactions in the tissues that protect against infections and wounds.

However, the most sophisticated, dynamic and effective defence is provided by cells that have developed special abilities to recognise and remove potentially dangerous substances. Some of these defence cells circulate continuously around the body in the blood, while others act as sentinels and are stationed in internal tissues or on the surface of the body to wait for foreign intruders.

# INNATE IMMUNITY

The first obstacles that an invasive pathogen meets are the body's physical barriers (Fig. 1). The initial and most obvious body barrier is the skin, which prevents pathogenic organisms from entering the body. When this barrier is breached, it heals rapidly to ensure that defence remains intact. However, pathogens that are transmitted by insect bites can penetrate the skin. The skin has other mechanisms, as well as the physical barrier itself, to prevent pathogens from entering, such as an acid pH and a high concentration of salts, which prevent pathogen colonisation. The fat secreted by sebaceous glands in the skin also contains various microbicides. For the mucosae, the presence of cilia and mucus prevent pathogens from penetrating these surfaces. There are also many antimicrobial agents in body secretions, such as gastric secretions in the stomach, and lysozyme in the saliva. Finally, the normal flora on the skin and in the gut also prevents colonisation by foreign agents by competing for the same ecological niche. These natural barriers are also called immune barriers.

If a pathogenic organism has been able to escape the immune barriers, it will encounter a second defensive barrier, the innate immune system (Fig. 1).

> The nonspecific or innate response is the body's first defensive barrier. It does not require prior sensitisation and is triggered in the hours immediately after an attack.

**Figure 1.** Immune barriers and the innate immune system.

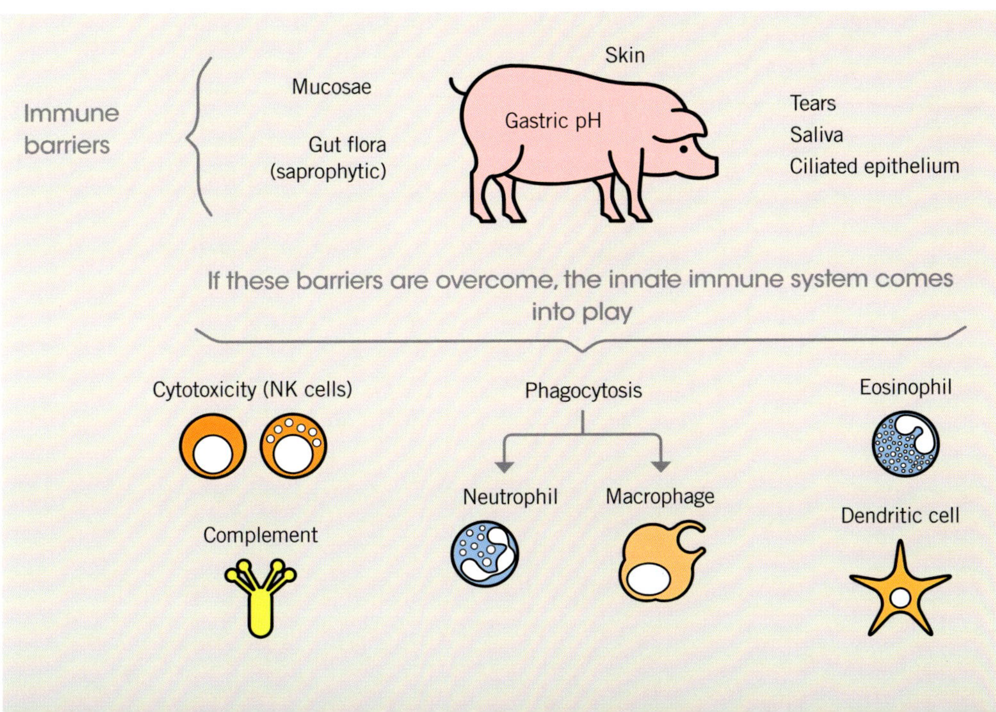

The innate immune response is based on the chemical differences between pathogenic organisms and components of the host's own body. This response consists of all the mechanisms triggered the moment a foreign agent (the pathogen itself or a product of the pathogen) enters, and it produces a danger signal within the body. Innate immune responses are characterised by being very fast and by lacking immunological memory (Fig. 2). Their main objective is to target and stop pathogen colonisation, by causing an inflammatory process. The process of inflammation involves heat, pain, redness, and swelling in the affected area. Figure 3 shows a simplified diagram of the inflammatory process. Two components of the innate immune system are involved in bringing about the inflammatory process: cellular and humoral components (Fig. 2 and Table 1).

**Figure 2.** Diagram of the acquired and innate immune responses.

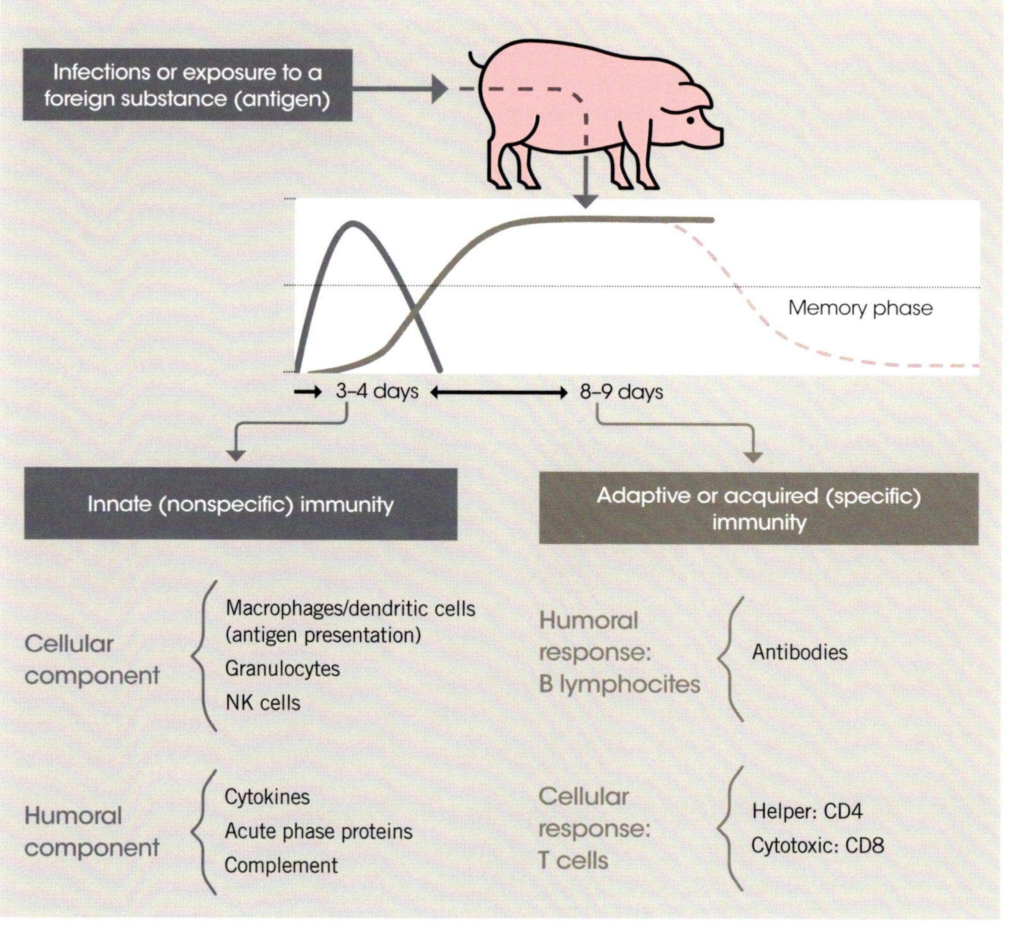

Figure 3. Most infectious agents induce an inflammatory response by activating the innate immune system (adapted from Murphy et al., 2001).

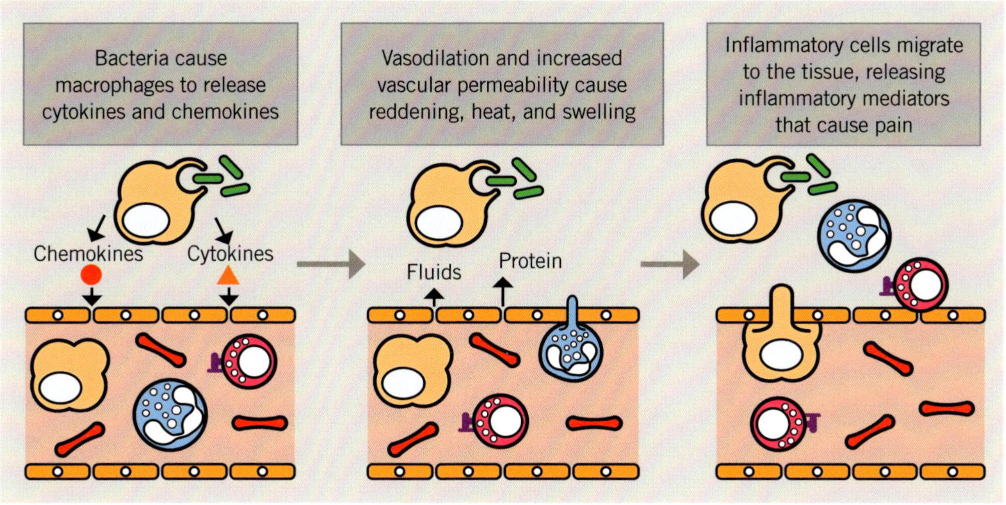


Table 1. Components and general functions of the innate immune system.

| Cellular components | |
|---|---|
| **Cell** | **Function** |
| Macrophage | ■ Phagocytosis and activation of antibacterial mechanisms<br>■ APC |
| Dendritic cell | ■ Peripheral antigen capture<br>■ Cytokine secretion<br>■ APC |
| Neutrophil | ■ Phagocytosis and activation of antibacterial mechanisms |
| NK | ■ Cellular cytotoxicity |
| Eosinophil | ■ Destruction of antibody-coated parasites |
| Basophil | ■ Unknown |
| Mast cell | ■ Release of activator granules |
| **Humoral components** | |
| **Proteins** | **Function** |
| Complement | ■ Activates the immune response<br>■ Facilitates phagocytosis<br>■ Organises cell lysis |
| Acute phase proteins | ■ Binding of complement proteins<br>■ Opsonisation |
| Cytokines | ■ Regulate cell functions, such as inflammation, chemotaxis, and the antiviral and antitumour response |

## CELLULAR COMPONENT

When a pathogen crosses the epithelial barrier and starts to replicate in host tissue, the first immune system cells that it encounters are usually phagocytic cells derived from the mononuclear phagocytic system. These cells continuously mature and enter the blood stream as monocytes, which may then migrate as macrophages to various tissues of the body, including the gastrointestinal tract, lungs, liver, and spleen. Macrophages also function as antigen-presenting cells (APCs). The second group of phagocytic cells that a pathogen comes into contact with is the neutrophils (polymorphs), which are found in the blood but not in the tissues. Both cell types can recognise, ingest, and destroy many pathogens without any further help from the immune system. Eosinophils, basophils, mast cells, and natural killer (NK) cells also form part of this nonspecific response (Table 1).

**Figure 4.** Innate immunity and pathogens.

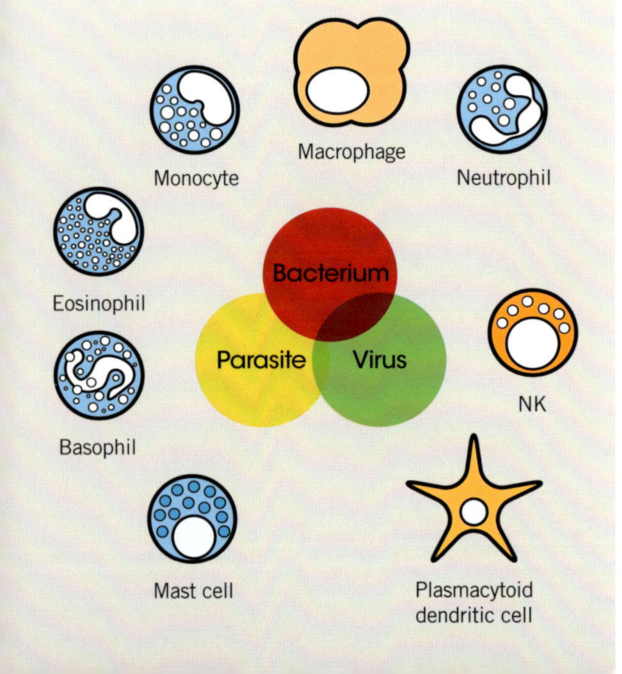


Innate immune system cells are characterised by being activated as soon as a foreign substance enters the body, for example after an injury. In such a case, all these cells move towards this focus, where they recognise and come into contact with the foreign substance. They destroy this by a process of phagocytosis and natural cytotoxicity. These cells are specialised in the recognition of certain pathogens, as shown in Figure 4.

Phagocytosis is the main element involved in this type of immune response. It is carried out in several stages: approach, phagocytosis, and lysis. Special mention should be made of the dendritic cells, APCs that secrete humoral innate immune system components. They have also specialised to capture foreign substances or small pathogen fragments (antigens) at the body's entry sites, where they act as sentinels. They then transport the antigenic material to the lymphatic organs, where they activate adaptive immune system cells. The main function of these cells is to form a link between the innate and adaptive immune systems (Fig. 5). Dendritic cells are very important, and their mode of activation can significantly influence the type of adaptive response that can be generated, which will be described later.

The main problem facing the immune system is how to recognise foreign substances (antigens) and differentiate them from the body's own structures. It also has to detect whether an antigen is harmful or not. In this case, the cells possess receptors for pathogen-associated molecular patterns (PAMPs) to recognise antigens. These receptors recognise patterns in the pathogen's repeated and conserved nucleic acid sequences and other molecules that are not found in the host. These include molecules which remain after microbial metabolism, like lipopolysaccharide (LPS), which is part of the bacterial wall.

> To conclude, the cellular components of the innate immune system can be summarised as macrophages, neutrophils, NK cells, eosinophils, basophils, mast cells, and dendritic cells. All of these cells specialise in the recognition of viruses, bacteria and parasites.

Figure 5. Mechanisms that protect against infection (adapted from Murphy et al., 2008).

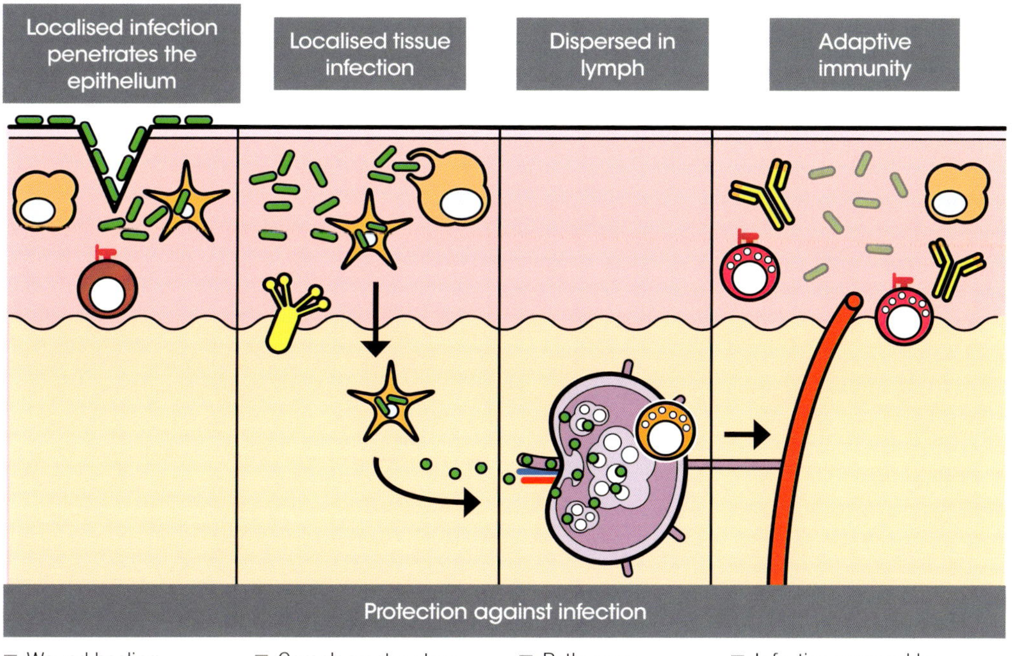


**Localised infection penetrates the epithelium**
- Wound healing.
- Antimicrobial proteins and peptides, phagocytes, and the complement system destroy invasive microorganisms.
- γδ T cell activation?

**Localised tissue infection**
- Complement system activation.
- Dendritic cells migrate to the lymph nodes.
- Phagocytosis.
- NK cell activation.
- Cytokine and chemokine production.

**Dispersed in lymph**
- Pathogens trapped and phagocytosed in the lymphatic tissue.
- Adaptive immunity starts with migration of dendritic cells.

**Adaptive immunity**
- Infection removed by specific antibodies, activation of the macrophages that depend on B cells and cytotoxic T cells.

## HUMORAL COMPONENT

Proteins and biochemical mediators which have various functions are included in this class (Table 1). The complement system is one of these groups of proteins, formed from a wide variety of proteins that are found in high levels in the plasma. The various components of the complement system are a set of plasma molecules that interact in a certain order to perform their role in the body's defence. Their function is to boost the inflammatory response, enable phagocytosis, and organise cellular lysis. Other proteins involved in this response are the acute phase proteins. These include some very important proteins, such as the pentraxin family, which includes C-reactive protein, serum amyloid protein, haptoglobin, and mannose-binding lectin (MBL). Their functions are varied, but they all bind and activate complement proteins, enabling opsonisation. Opsonisation can proceed in two ways: antibody opsonisation is the process by which a pathogen is marked with an antibody for ingestion and destruction by a phagocyte. The cell can also be destroyed by a process called antibody-dependent cytotoxicity, where the pathogen does not have to be phagocytosed to be destroyed.

The last, large family of proteins activated in the innate immune response is the cytokines. These proteins regulate the function of the cells that produce them, or the function of other types of cell. They are responsible for intercellular communication, and they activate specific membrane receptors. They also regulate cell proliferation and differentiation, chemotaxis and growth, and they modulate immunoglobulin secretion. Immunoglobulins are mainly produced by activated lymphocytes and macrophages, although they can also be secreted by other cells. Their main activity is to regulate inflammation. Some cytokines are pro-inflammatory (TNF-$\alpha$, IL-1), and others are anti-inflammatory (IL-2, IL-4). One very important group of cytokines are type I interferons (IFN-alpha, beta, omega, epsilon, and kappa) which are produced naturally by most animals' immune systems in response to external agents. Interferon production is triggered by other cytokines, such as IL-1, IL-2 and TNF-$\alpha$, which are synthesised when a virus is detected in the body.

In conclusion, the humoral components of the innate immune system can be summarised as complement system proteins, acute phase proteins, and cytokines (Table 1). The nonspecific defence mechanisms provide a good system of protection, but they are often insufficient to defend the body effectively. Fortunately, the body also has a specific immune response, termed adaptive or acquired (Fig. 2).

# ADAPTIVE (ACQUIRED) IMMUNITY

Any pathogens that manage to evade innate immune system mechanisms are met with a defence system that specifically recognises and destroys invading agents. This system is highly specialised, but it takes several days, or longer, to become functional (Table 2, Fig. 2). Antigen specificity is acquired, and enables responses that are adapted to specific pathogens or to cells infected with these pathogens. The adaptive immune response begins when an APC (often a dendritic cell) captures a pathogen in an infected tissue and migrates through the lymph system to the peripheral lymph nodes, where it interacts with lymphocytes. This dendritic cell thus forms a bridge between the innate and adaptive immune systems (Fig. 5).

The main cells of the adaptive immune system are B cells and T cells. Both are derived from multipotent haematopoietic stem cells in the bone marrow. Figure 6 is a diagram of how all the cell types that have been described so far, involved in both innate and adaptive immunity, are generated.

B cells are involved in the humoral immune response (humoral component), while T cells are mainly involved in the cell-mediated immune response (cellular component).

Lymphocytes are mostly found in the lymphatic organs, blood, and mucosae. Although the lymphocyte population appears to be homogeneous, it is actually diverse and heterogeneous. They are not differentiated by structure, but by some characteristic receptors

Table 2. Comparison of the innate and adaptive immune systems.

| Mechanisms | Innate | Adaptive |
|---|---|---|
| Cellular components | Macrophages, dendritic cells, NK cells, etc. | T and B cells |
| Humoral components | Complement, acute phase proteins, and cytokines | Antibodies |
| Evolutionary history | Ancient (found in nearly all life forms) | Recent (only found in more evolved life forms) |
| Activation | Rapid (minutes to hours) | Slow (days to weeks) |
| Specificity | Common repetitive pathogenic molecule structures | Unique antigens |
| Memory | None | Yes |
| Efficacy | No | Improves with exposure to the pathogen |

Figure 6. All blood cells, including lymphocytes, originate from germ cells in the haematopoietic system, which is located in the bone marrow (adapted from Murphy et al., 2005).

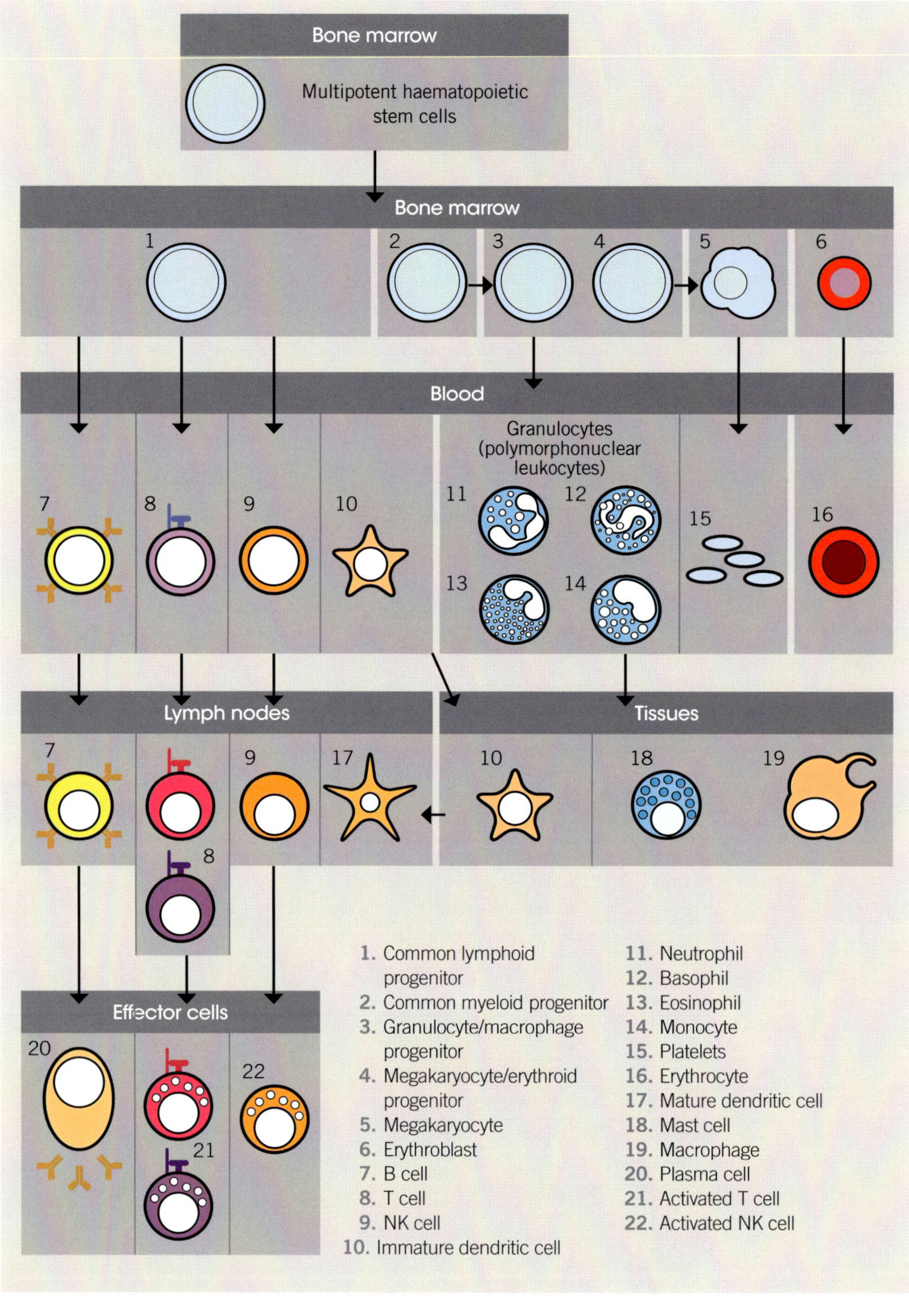

on their membranes, and by their function. The pattern of the receptors on each cell is called the immunophenotype, and lymphocyte subpopulations can be differentiated by this pattern. Each receptor molecule on the cell surface has a name which refers to its function and/or chemical structure, and a name formed by the letters CD (cluster of differentiation) followed by a number (e.g. CD4).

The CD molecules expressed on the surface of cells in domestic animals can be split into two categories: molecules which have their counterpart in the human and/or mouse, and so have the same name, and heterologous molecules. The latter are named using the initials WC (workshops cluster) preceded by an abbreviation for the species concerned (e.g. SWC8: swine WC8).

Figure 7. Most common surface receptors on B cells (a) and T cells (b), their ligands, and general functions.

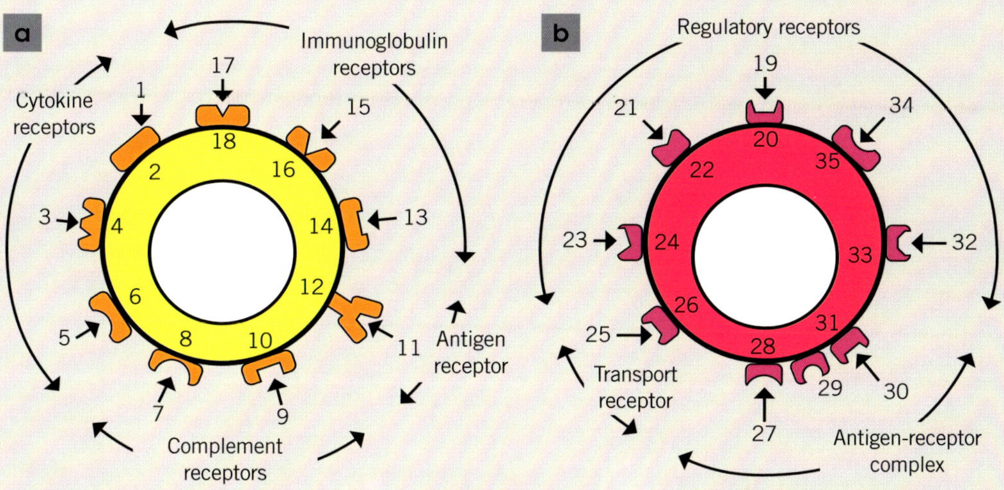


1. IL-5
2. CD125
3. IL-4
4. CD124
5. IL-2
6. CD25/CD122
7. Complement
8. CD35
9. Complement
10. CD21
11. Antigen
12. BCR
13. IgE
14. CD23
15. IgG
16. CD32
17. IgM
18. FcµR
19. Histamine
20. H3
21. Immunoglobulins
22. FcR
23. Complement
24. CD35
25. Transferrin
26. CD71
27. MHC molecules
28. CD4 or CD8
29. CD3
30. Antigen
31. TCR
32. CD58
33. CD2
34. IL-2
35. CD25

B and T cells both contain receptor molecules which recognise specific structures (Fig. 7). T cells generally recognise a foreign body, such as a pathogen, after the antigens have been processed and presented in combination with a receptor on one of the body's own cells. This receptor molecule is called a major histocompatibility complex (MHC). MHC molecules comprise a family of proteins, notably class I and class II MHC. Although molecules in class I and class II are functionally different, there are characteristic structural similarities that are highly relevant to peptide bonding and to recognition by T cells.

All MHC molecules have four segments: one segment for peptide binding (the cleft), one immunoglobulin (Ig)-type domain, a transmembrane segment, and a carboxy-terminus cytoplasmic portion (Fig. 8). The polymorphic (variable) sector of an MHC molecule is located in the peptide-binding cleft. Amino acids which vary from one allele to another are found around this cleft, generating the polymorphism which characterises an MHC. An MHC can deal with a wide range of antigens due to this high degree of variability in the peptide-binding region. Class I MHC molecules are present in a constantly active state in all nucleated cells within the body. Class II MHC molecules are only present in antigen-presenting cells. B cells, macrophages and, predominantly, dendritic cells are found in this cell group.

There are two main T cell subtypes: the killer or cytotoxic T cell, and the helper T cell (Th). Cytotoxic T cells only recognise antigens bound to class I MHC molecules. Once these lymphocytes recognise the antigen peptides presented by class I molecules, they become activated and lyse the cell infected by the endogenous microorganism. However, helper T cells only recognise antigens bound

**Figure 8.** The four key immune system antigen receptors (TCR, class I MHC, class II MHC, and BCR) are constructed using immunoglobulin domains as essential elements. Each of these is bound to the antigen by their different domains, and they are all members of the immunoglobulin superfamily (adapted from Tizard, 2013).

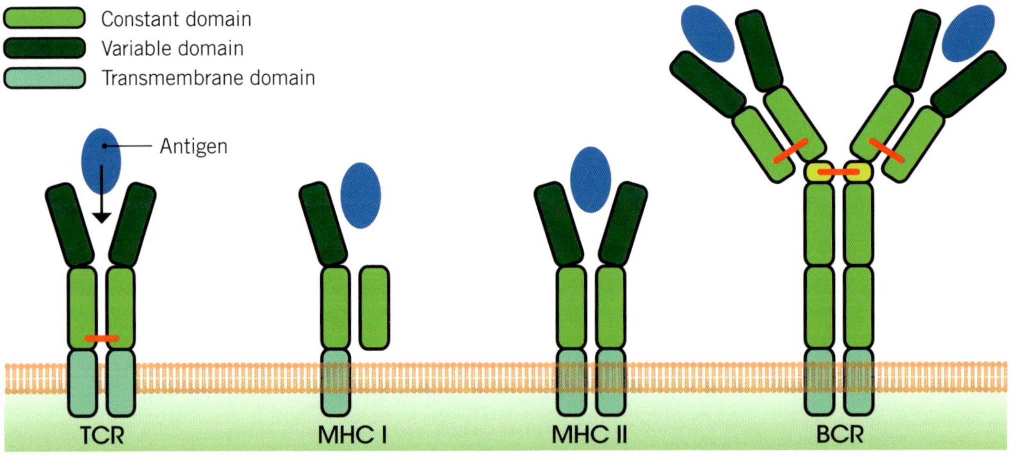

**Figure 9.** Role of CD4 and CD8 in promoting T cell-mediated response. These molecules bind the T cell to the APC, joining the cells together and ensuring that an effective signal is transmitted between them (adapted from Tizard, 2013).

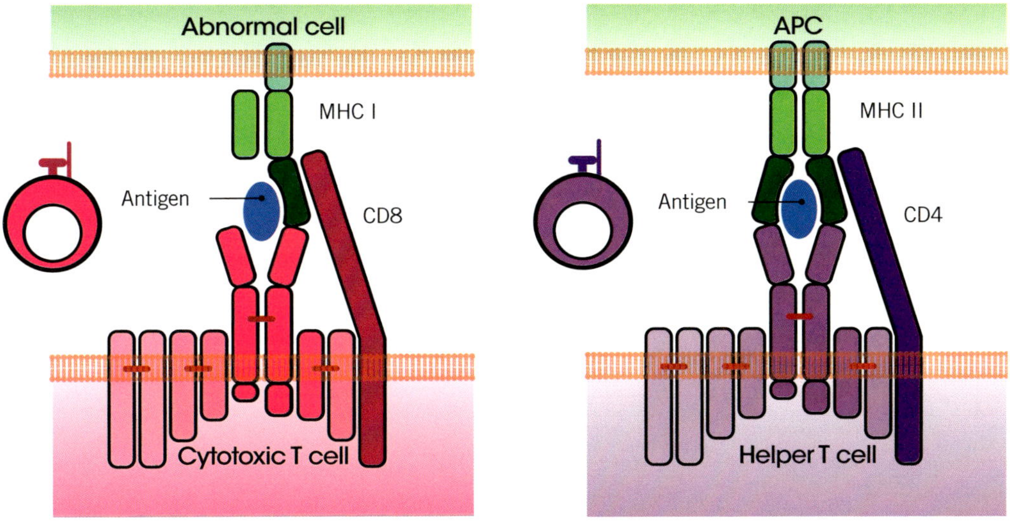


to class II MHC molecules. These two mechanisms of antigen presentation reflect the different roles of the two different types of lymphocyte (Fig. 9). A third subtype is made up of $\gamma\delta$ T cells (gamma delta T cells) which recognise intact antigens that have not been bound to MHC receptors. This is why this cell type is associated more with the innate than the adaptive immune system.

However, the specific B cell antigen receptor is an antibody molecule on the surface of the B cell (Fig. 8) which recognises whole pathogens without the need for the antigens to be processed beforehand. Each B cell line expresses a different antibody on their surface, so the totality of the B cell antigen receptors in the body represents all the antibodies that the body is able to manufacture.

In general terms, the adaptive immune system is divided into two, according to the different responses that occur when a pathogenic agent is recognised: some pathogens enter the body through body fluids, where they grow and multiply. In these cases, the antibody-mediated response is the most efficient. However, others grow inside the cells and cannot be accessed by antibodies, so cell-mediated action is essential.

> Humoral immunity is normally understood to be a response mediated by antibodies secreted by B cells, and cellular immunity comprises the actions mediated by T cells (cooperation, cytokine production, and cytotoxicity).

## HUMORAL COMPONENT

The B cell identifies a pathogen when the antibodies on its surface bind to specific foreign antigens. Each B cell is covered with between 200,000 and 500,000 antigen receptors termed B-cell receptors (BCRs) (Figs. 7–8). When the antigen–antibody complex moves inside the B cell, it is processed by proteolysis and broken down into peptides. The B cell then presents these peptide antigens on its surface, bound to class II MHC molecules. This MHC–antigen combination sometimes attracts a helper T cell with receptors that match this MHC–antigen complex. The T cell then releases cytokines, activating B cells. At other times, B cells are activated without the assistance of helper T cells when they simply recognise the antigen in body fluids. Once a B cell has been activated, it starts to divide, and its progeny secrete millions of copies of the antibody that recognises that particular antigen. These antibodies circulate in the blood plasma and lymph. They bind to the pathogens that carry those particular antigens, marking them for destruction through complement activation or phagocytosis. The antibodies can also neutralise some threats directly, by binding bacterial toxins or interfering with the receptors used by viruses and bacteria to infect cells.

## CELLULAR COMPONENT

T cells are a heterogeneous cell group with respect to their function, but all T cells have specific membrane receptors, termed T cell receptors (TCRs) (Figs. 9–10). Just like their equivalent in the B cells, these specific receptors are complex structures made up of various proteins. Two large subpopulations can be identified within the T cell group, classified according to the structure of their TCRs: the receptor in one group is made up of α and β chains, and the other group γ and δ chains. The latter are called γδ T cells. The function of the TCR is to transmit a signal to a cell once it has bound to an antigen, informing the cell of this occurrence.

γδ T cells represent a small subpopulation of T cells where the antigenic molecules that stimulate them are largely unknown. However, these lymphocytes are peculiar in that they appear not to need the antigens to be processed and presented bound to MHC molecules. γδ T cells are also thought to play a major part in the recognition of lipid antigens. These cells fall somewhere between the innate and adaptive systems, due to their diverse functions. Their functions, and relative levels circulating in the blood, also differ in the various mammalian species.

A protein called CD3 is included in the αβ T cell antigen–recognition complex and this is used as a marker for all αβ T cells (Fig. 9). T cells also have other surface markers that differentiate their functions and identify their phenotype. CD4 and CD8 are important ones. CD4 is only found in T helper cells, and it characterises cells that recognise antigens bound to class II MHC in APCs. Conversely, CD8 is only found in the cytotoxic T cells that attack and destroy infected or tumour cells. These are the killer T cells. The CD8 molecule is a coreceptor for the bond between the TCR and class I MHC (Fig. 9).

Cytotoxic T cells are a subgroup of the $CD8^+$ αβ T cells that destroy cells infected by viruses (and other pathogens), or are infected or damaged by other means. As with

Figure 10. Major differences between Th1 and Th2 cell populations. Note that they are triggered by different costimulatory signals and they secrete a different combination of cytokines (adapted from Tizard, 2013).

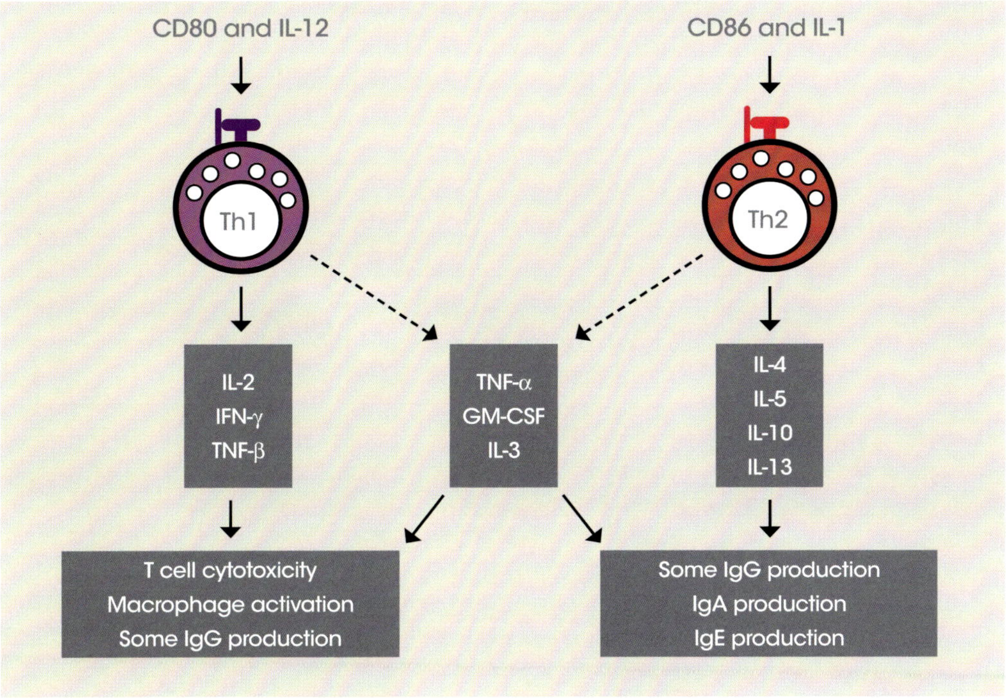


B cells, each type of T cell recognises a different antigen. Cytotoxic T cells are activated when their TCR receptor recognises a specific antigen bound to a complex on a class I MHC receptor of another cell. Cytotoxins are then released and form pores in the plasma membrane of the target or receptor cell, allowing entry of ions, water and toxins (Fig. 9). This kills the target cell in a process called apoptosis. Death of the target cell, induced by cytotoxic T cells, is very important in preventing virus replication. T cell activation is also very strictly controlled, and it usually requires a very strong activation signal from the MHC–antigen complex, or additional activation signals from helper T cells.

> The proportions of $CD4^+$ and/or $CD8^+$ cells can be used to estimate immune system function, and thus indicate some kind of pathology.

Helper T cells (Th cells) help determine the type of adaptive response mounted by the body against a particular pathogen. These cells are not cytotoxic and do not directly destroy infected cells or pathogens, but they do control the immune response by directing other cells to carry out these tasks.

These lymphocytes possess a TCR on their surface that recognises antigens bound to the class II MHC molecules that have a CD4 molecule as coreceptor. Activation of a helper T cell causes it to release cytokines that affect the activity of many kinds of cell. Helper T cells include various subtypes classified according to the profile of the cytokines that they produce, and these can be grouped into Th1, Th2 and Th17 cells (Fig. 11). These subtypes have mainly been defined in mice and humans so they cannot be assumed to function in the same way in other mammals, including pigs.

In general, Th1 cells respond best to antigens presented by both myeloid dendritic cells and B cells, and they also need a costimulatory signal, in this case CD80. Myeloid dendritic cells also activate these Th1 cells by secreting IL-12 and IL-18 (Fig. 10). When stimulated, the Th1 cells mainly secrete IL-2 and IFN-γ, the functions of which are summarised in Figure 11. Basically, the cytokine signals released by Th1 cells boost the microbe

**Figure 11.** Cytokines produced by Th1 and Th2 cells, and their main properties (adapted from Tizard, 2013).

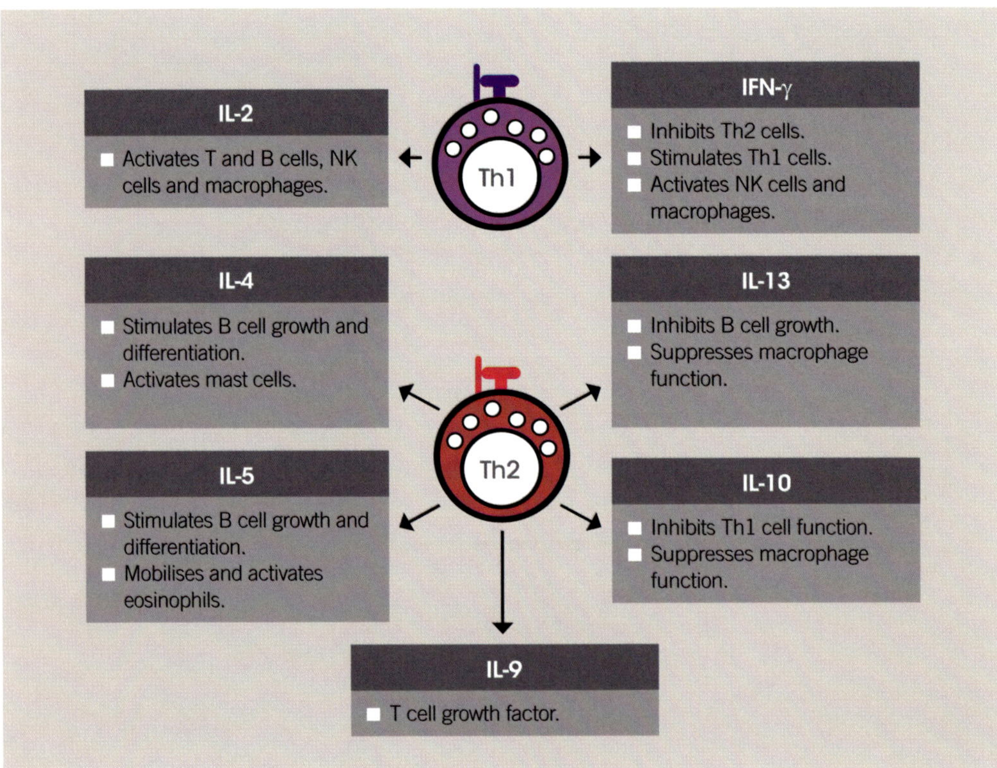

killing activities of macrophages and cytotoxic T cell activity, and increase production of a particular antibody isotype (IgG2). Generating this kind of response is very important in combating intracellular organisms.

Th2 cells respond to antigens presented by plasmacytoid dendritic cells and macrophages and, to a lesser extent, by B cells. These APCs secrete IL-1 (and IL-4), and also need a different costimulatory signal (CD86) to stimulate Th2 cells (Fig. 10). Once activated, Th2 cells secrete enough interleukins to up-regulate the molecules expressed on the surface of T cells and provide the additional stimulatory signals required to activate B cells, which can increase antibody production significantly, especially of the isotypes IgG1 and IgGE. They can also stimulate mast cells, and mobilise and activate eosinophils.

Conversely, IFN-γ (interleukin typical of a Th1 response) inhibits Th2 cell function (Fig. 12). A typical example of this is inhibition of the Th1 response in pregnant females, to maintain gestation and prevent abortion. Different antigens can stimulate these Th cell subpopulations in different ways, so the T cell response to *Toxocara canis* antigens is of the Th2 type, as IL-4 and IL-5 are the main secretions (Fig. 12), while T cells exposed to purified protein derivative (PPD), an antigen of *Mycobacterium tuberculosis* trigger a Th1 response, where IL-2 and IFN-γ are the main secretions.

It should be noted that an increased Th1 response reduces the Th2 response, so it is impossible to increase both responses at the same time, as some of the interleukins most relevant to the Th2 response (IL-10 and IL-13) reduce Th1 cell and macrophage activity.

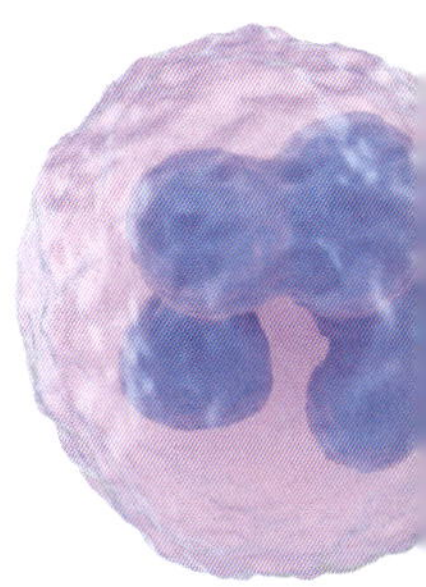

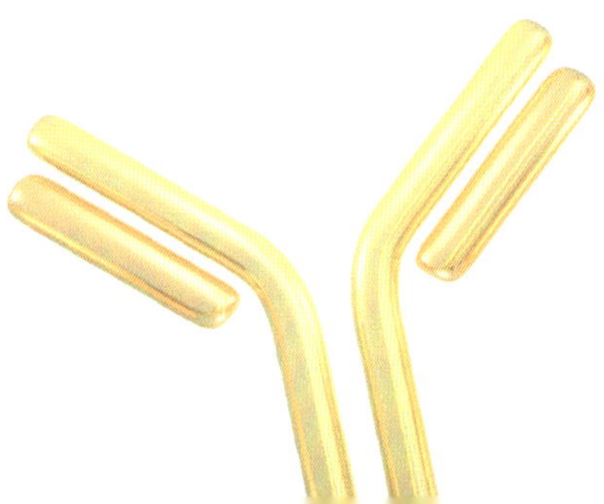

**Figure 12.** Different antigens lead to the creation of different Th cell subpopulations. For example, T cells exposed to a *Toxocara canis* nematode parasite antigen induce a Th2 response and secrete mainly IL-4 and IL-5. Conversely, when T cells are exposed to PPD, an antigen of *Mycobacterium tuberculosis*, they trigger a Th1 response characterised by IFN-γ and IL-2 secretion (adapted from Tizard, 2013).

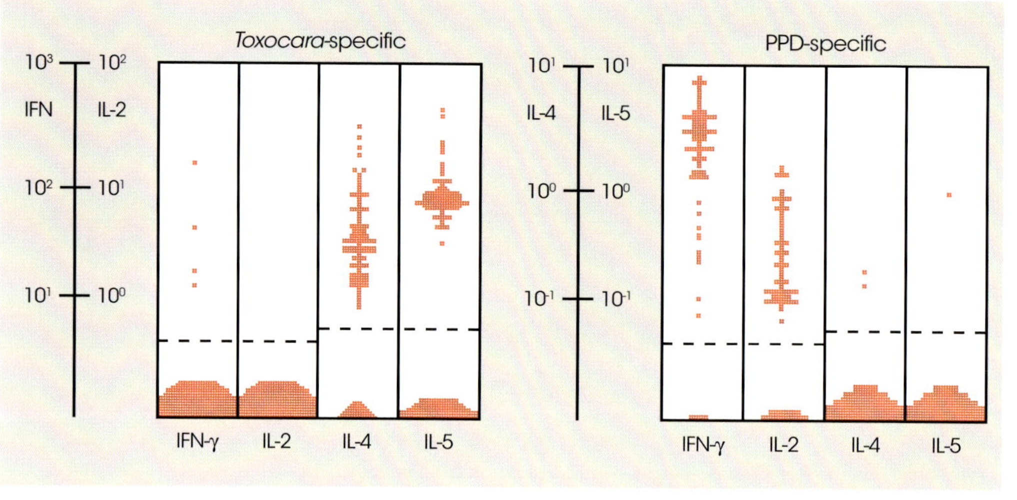


## DYNAMICS OF THE IMMUNE RESPONSE

Vertebrates resist infection by pathogenic microorganisms in various ways. First, they prevent them from entering their bodies. At this point they should be controlled by the immune barrier but, if the immune barrier is overcome, the innate immune system will intervene, normally controlling and removing the infection completely, or controlling it until the adaptive immune system comes into play. The innate immune system's ability to respond is immediate and develops in the days immediately after infection. The third and final phase of the immune response is the adaptive phase, which requires several days before it starts to develop. The dynamics of the immune response are summarised in Table 3, which shows the three phases described above and the various types of pathogens that the animal might encounter.

The adaptive immune system can 'remember' an antigen and learn how to destroy it so that the defence system is activated even faster if the pathogen reappears. This process is called immunological memory. In this system, the more the body encounters a pathogen, the more effective the defensive measures develop to destroy it (Fig. 13).

Table 3. Dynamics of the immune response according to the type of pathogen involved (adapted from Murphy et al., 2008).

| | Stages of the immune response | | |
|---|---|---|---|
| | Immediate (0–4 hours) | Early (4–96 hours) | Late (96–100 hours) |
| | ■ Nonspecific<br>■ Innate<br>■ No memory<br>■ Nonspecific T cells | ■ Nonspecific + antigen-specific<br>■ Induced<br>■ No memory<br>■ Nonspecific T cells | ■ Specific<br>■ Induced<br>■ Memory<br>■ Antigen-specific T cells |
| Barrier functions | ■ Skin, epithelium | ■ Local inflammation (C5a)<br>■ Local TN-α | ■ IgA antibodies in body cavities<br>■ IgE antibodies in mast cells<br>■ Local inflammation |
| Response to extracellular pathogens | ■ Phagocytes<br>■ Alternative complement and MBL pathway | ■ MBL<br>■ C-reactive protein<br>■ Antibodies from B cells, independent of T cells<br>■ Complement | ■ IgG antibodies and Fc receptor-bearing cells<br>■ IgG and IgM antibodies + classical complement pathway |
| Response to intracellular bacteria | ■ Macrophages | ■ Activation of macrophages dependent on activated NK cells<br>■ IL-1, IL-6, TNF-α, IL-12 | ■ Activation of macrophage T cells by IFN-γ |
| Response to cells infected by viruses | ■ NK cells | ■ IFN-α and IFN-β<br>■ NK cells activated by IL-12 | ■ Cytotoxic T cells<br>■ IFN-γ |

Figure 13. Immunological memory (adapted from Murphy et al., 2005).

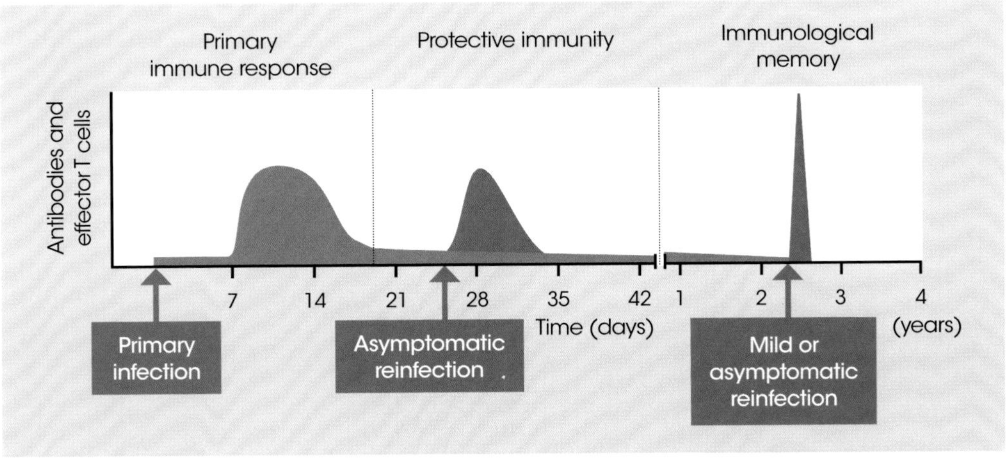

This type of response is obvious when antibody production by an individual challenged by a pathogen, or by repeated doses of a vaccine, is quantified. So, in secondary responses, or responses to antigen challenges, antibodies in the body will bind to the antigen whenever it is introduced, and APCs will present it to be processed effectively (Fig. 14). Memory B cells can also recognise a specific antigen and start a process of proliferation which increases the antibody titre significantly.

The body's ability to produce a specific response is maintained by these memory cells. If a pathogen infects an organism more than once, these memory cells recognise it and trigger a specific response to eliminate it quickly. When B and/or T cells are activated and start to divide, some of their progeny are converted into long-lived memory cells, and the rest are removed. Throughout the animal's lifetime, these cells remember each particular pathogen that they meet and they can trigger a strong response if they detect that specific pathogen again. This process is called adaptive because it occurs throughout the lifetime of the individual as an adaptation to infection by that particular pathogen, and it ensures the immune system is prepared for future challenges. Immunological memory can be passive and short-term, or active and long-term. Vaccines rely on generating a long-term immunological memory.

**Figure 14.** Dynamics of the antibody response to various challenges by the same antigen (adapted from Murphy et al., 2008).

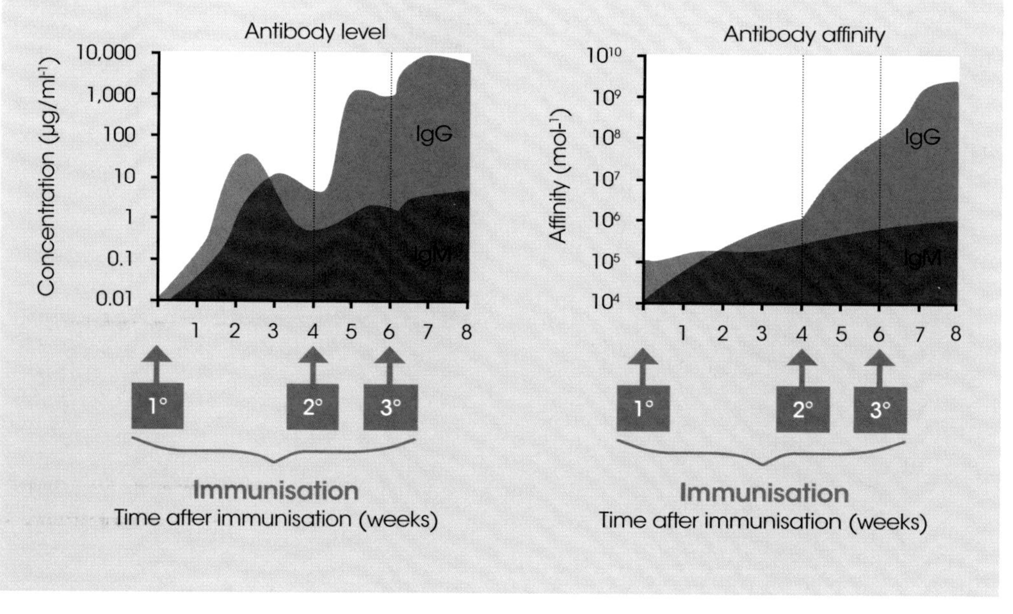

## RELATIVE IMPORTANCE OF CELLULAR AND HUMORAL IMMUNITY IN EFFECTIVE PROTECTION

Many pathogens trigger both cellular and humoral adaptive immune responses, and the two are often needed to control infection and build up good immune protection, although the relative importance of the effector mechanisms and the different types of antibodies generated vary according to the pathogens involved. The importance of cytotoxic T cells in the destruction of cells infected by viruses has been previously discussed, but the importance of antibodies in removing viruses should not be overlooked. The cellular form of immune response is critical to destroy cells infected by intracellular pathogens. Conversely, the humoral immune response is essential to control infections by extracellular bacteria. In fact, IgG and IgM antibodies mark out bacteria and make them more susceptible to phagocytosis. Ideally, for each species of animal, we should confirm the best type of adaptive response needed to generate protective immunity to their most common pathogens. More detailed information is available for human diseases, and Table 4 shows the roles of humoral and cellular immunity in protecting against some of these. The information available on pigs is discussed in Chapter 3.

Table 4. The immune system uses various mechanisms to protect against reinfection. The table below shows the roles of humoral and cellular immunity in controlling infections caused by viruses, fungi, parasites, and intracellular and extracellular bacteria. The colours red (highly relevant), yellow (slightly relevant) and white (not relevant) indicate the role played in protection. Paler colours indicate that the protective role is not known with any certainty. Note: the CD4 T response in this table indicates only those involved in macrophage activation (adapted from Murphy et al., 2008).

| | | | Humoral immunity | | | | Cellular immunity | |
|---|---|---|---|---|---|---|---|---|
| | Infectious agent | Disease | IgM | IgG | IgE | IgA | CD4 T cells | CD8 T cells |
| Virus | Herpes zoster virus | Chickenpox | | | | | | |
| | Epstein–Barr virus | Mononucleosis | | | | | | |
| | Flu virus | Flu | | | | | | |
| | Polio virus | Poliomyelitis | | | | | | |
| Intracellular bacteria | *Rickettsia prowazekii* | Typhus | | | | | | |
| | Mycobacteria | Tuberculosis, leprosy | | | | | | |
| Extracellular bacteria | *Staphylococcus aureus* | Furunculosis | | | | | | |
| | *Streptococcus pneumonia* | Pneumonia | | | | | | |
| | *Neisseria meningitidis* | Meningitis | | | | | | |
| | *Corynebacterium diphtheriae* | Diphtheria | | | | | | |
| | *Vibrio cholerae* | Cholera | | | | | | |
| Fungi | *Candida albicans* | Candidiasis | | | | | | |
| Protozoa | *Plasmodium* spp. | Malaria | | | | | | |
| | *Trypanosoma* spp. | Trypanosomiasis | | | | | | |
| Trematodes | Schistosomes | Schistosomiasis | | | | | | |

# 02

# GENERAL PRINCIPLES OF VACCINES AND VACCINATION

# GENERAL PRINCIPLES OF VACCINES AND VACCINATION

## INTRODUCTION

The basic objective in animal production is to obtain high quality protein that is totally safe for the consumer. To meet this objective, animals from an appropriate gene pool should be used, and they should be housed in suitable facilities, fed on a diet that is suitable for their species and age, and be free from disease at slaughter. Animals can obviously suffer from diseases throughout their productive cycle, and these can arise from various sources, although those caused by bacteria, viruses and parasites are the most common. Preventive medicine is used to try to reduce the negative effects of these diseases; more specifically, preventive medicine is the branch of veterinary science that studies disease prevention, and the maintenance of animal health and production at optimum levels of profitability. A combination of sanitary and medical measures can be used (Fig. 1). Although the objective of this chapter is not to describe sanitary measures in depth, their importance should not be overlooked.

**Figure 1.** Disease control measures.

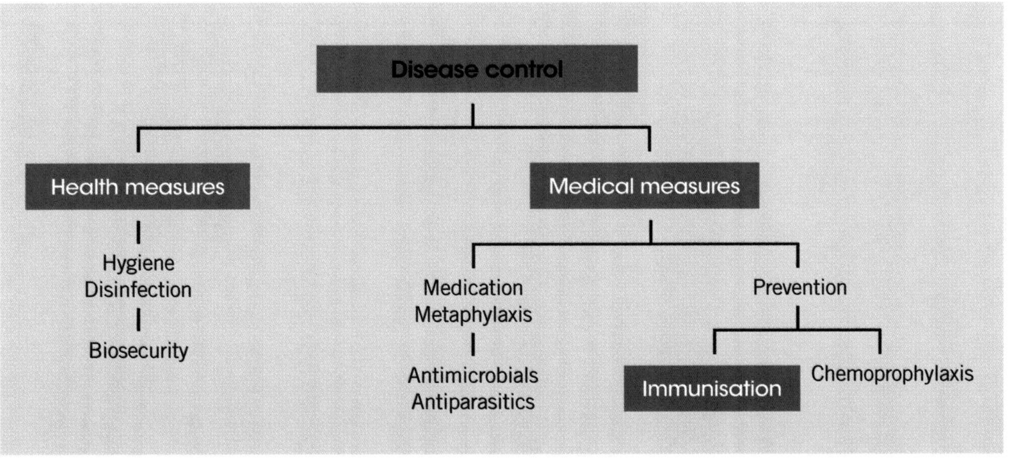

Hygiene and disinfection measures are essential for disease control on the farm, as they significantly reduce the potential to acquire new diseases by reducing the number of pathogens in the environment to below the minimum infective dose (the quantity of a microorganism needed for animals to be infected).

Medical measures, on the other hand, comprise the attempt to prevent disease from occurring, to keep a disease under control, to treat animals for a disease that they already have, and/or reduce the negative effects of the disease once acquired (Fig. 1). Therapeutic treatment, metaphylaxis and prophylaxis can all be used in animals:

- Therapy deals with curing a sick animal. In Figure 1, this corresponds to the use of antimicrobials or antiparasitics to cure diseases caused by bacteria or parasites respectively.
- Metaphylaxis consists of applying medical measures to the whole animal population, even though only some are showing signs of disease. This decision is taken when there is considered to be a very high risk of many animals in the group becoming ill if the prevalence of the disease reaches a certain level. In Figure 1, this entails the administration of antimicrobials and antiparasitics to the whole animal population (e.g. the whole farm), although only some of them may actually have the disease.
- Finally, prophylactic measures are used to prevent a disease appearing in a population. In this case, there are no sick animals at the time of implementing these measures. As shown in Figure 1, prophylaxis can be based on medicating the animals or trying to acquire immunity against the disease to be prevented. The use of drugs for prophylactic purposes is very controversial, especially antimicrobials, so it should be avoided wherever possible. It is therefore becoming more and more accepted that prophylaxis in animal populations should be based on acquiring and/or boosting good immunity.

As mentioned in the first chapter, immunity can be innate or acquired. Innate immunity has no memory and is not directed at a particular pathogen.

Preventative medicine is based on increasing acquired immunity to a variety of pathogens, as this type of immunity is specific and is retained in memory.

Acquired immunity (Fig. 2) can be natural or artificial. Natural immunity can be acquired by the transfer of passive immunity from the mother to the offspring, or by developing and overcoming the disease. The next chapter of this book will be devoted to this transfer of passive immunity, as it is extremely important in some pig diseases. Animals can sometimes be exposed to pathogens in order to generate active immunity. This occurs during a stage of rearing that takes account of the epidemiological profile of the disease. However, this measure can be considered exceptional as it means that all the animals will contract the disease, which can have serious implications for animal welfare. Finally, artificial immunity can be passive or active. Passive artificial immunisation mainly involves the administration of antibodies, for example to prevent the development of a serious disease, such as tetanus. This approach is extremely uncommon in production animals. On the other hand, active artificial immunity is generated by administering vaccines, and this is very common.

Vaccination is one of the most effective ways to control infectious diseases in humans and animals.

There is no doubt that the eradication of human smallpox worldwide, and classical swine fever and Aujeszky's disease from some countries, would not have been possible without the systematic use of vaccination.

Figure 2. Types of acquired immunity.

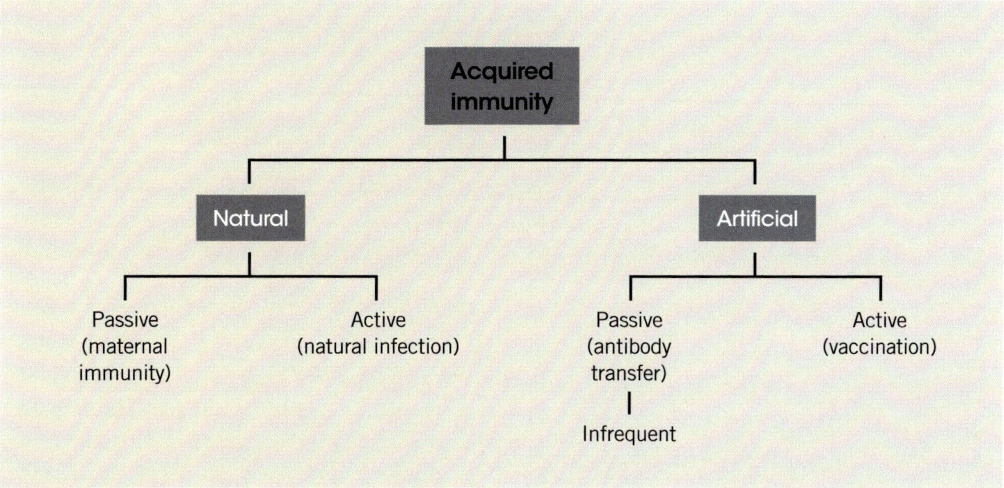

# METHODS OF ACTIVE ARTIFICIAL IMMUNISATION

Methods of active artificial immunisation are based on administering antigens to an individual in order to develop an immune response. Revaccination also generates a secondary immune response that is much more powerful than the primary response, as shown in Figure 3. The downside to this strategy is that protection is not conferred immediately after vaccination, as an effective immune response takes some time to develop. The characteristics of the ideal vaccine are summarised in Table 1. Unfortunately, an effective ability to provoke an immunogenic response is not possible without adverse reactions, so any vaccine involves a compromise between the advantages and disadvantages. From an antigen perspective, a vaccine can contain live organisms that can replicate themselves, or non-living (inactivated) organisms, or components of these, that cannot replicate. Figure 4 shows all the types of antigen, and methods used to acquire immunity, based on the classification mentioned above.

Although there are many technological possibilities, the vaccines that are most commonly available for pigs are inactivated vaccines (viral and bacterial), live vaccines (mainly viral, a few bacterial), and vaccines containing microorganism subunits (toxoids or fractions of microorganisms that generate a protective immune response).

All vaccines are composed of an antigen or a combination of antigens and other components, usually adjuvants. These are substances that mainly affect how the body responds to vaccination, and can potentiate or modify this response to the antigen (e.g. induce cellular immunity to an inactivated pathogen). Their use allows the amount of antigen required, or the number of doses administered, to be reduced, and they can be essential to induce long-term memory for soluble antigens. The exact mechanisms of how adjuvants act are not known but they can be classified into three general types:

- Depot: delayed antigen release at the vaccination site, prolonging the immune response.
- Particulate: improved antigen access to the antigen-presenting cells (APCs), optimising antigen presentation.
- Immunostimulatory: improved cytokine response and selective stimulation of the Th1 or Th2 response by appropriate costimulation.

Table 2 shows the most commonly used adjuvants and the type of Th1 or Th2 responses that they can encourage. Although more is being discovered every day about how adjuvants function, it is likely that the therapeutic margin between adjuvant efficacy and toxicity is narrow. This is because the mechanism for efficacy and toxicity is basically the same. For example, the physiological function of Toll-like receptors is to stimulate inflammation and the resulting immune response. Stimulating these receptors with certain adjuvants during

**Figure 3.** Vaccine functioning is based on immunological memory. This entails the development of an immune response that is faster and stronger than in previous encounters with the same antigen. It thus allows the immunised individual to resist reinfection when it comes into contact with that infectious agent again.

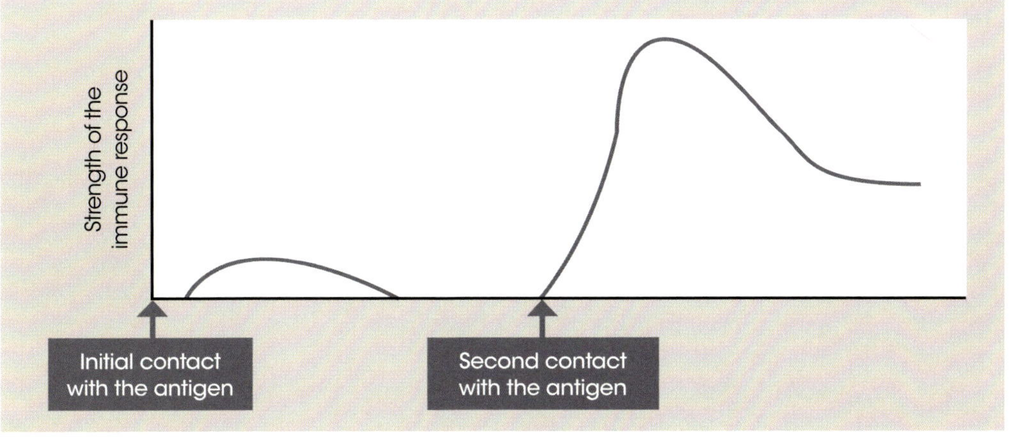


**Figure 4.** Types of acquired immunity and methods used to induce protection (adapted from Tizard, 2013).

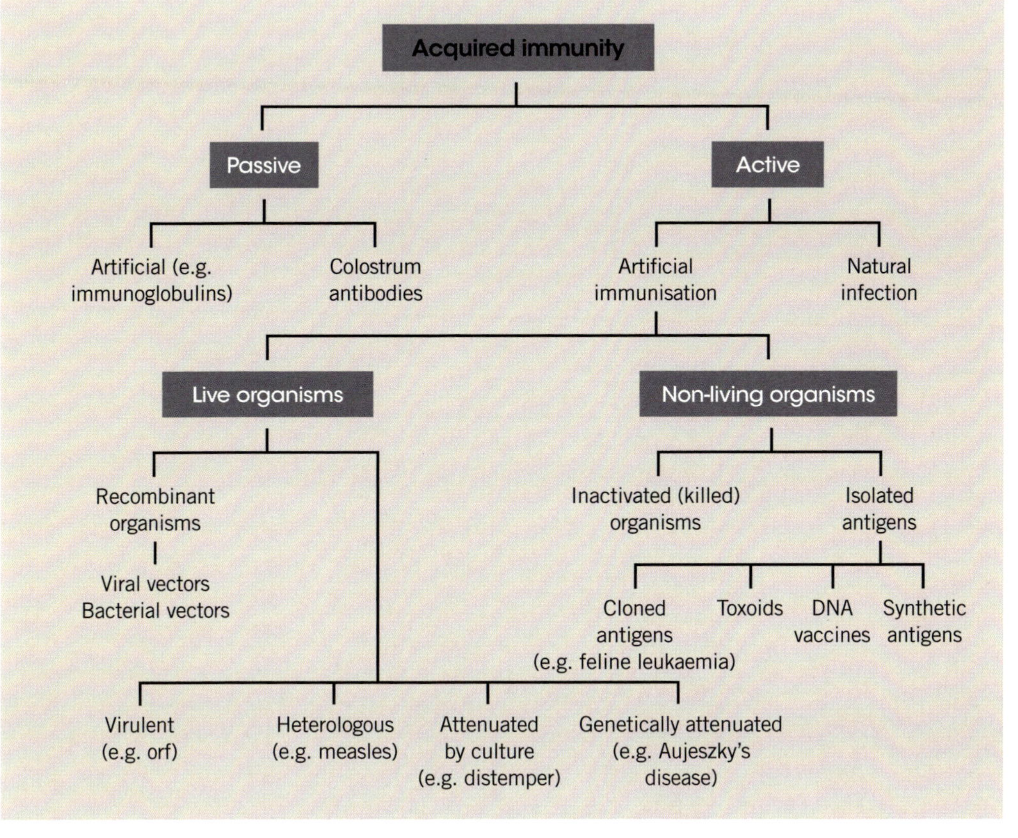

Table 1. Characteristics of the ideal vaccine.

| |
|---|
| Induces sterilising immunity for life |
| Induces cellular and humoral immunity |
| Needs only a single dose |
| Has no residual pathogenicity |
| Covers all types of a particular pathogen (i.e. is universal) |
| Does not cause adverse reactions |
| Is easy to produce |
| Is reasonably priced |
| Is easy to administer |
| Does not require special storage conditions |
| Enables differentiation between vaccinated and infected animals |

Table 2. Characteristics of the responses induced by the most common types of adjuvant. The arrows indicate a stronger (↑) or weaker (↓) response. More plus signs (+) indicate a stronger effect with this adjuvant.

| Type of adjuvant | | Th1 response | Th2 response |
|---|---|---|---|
| Aluminium hydroxide | Depot (+) | ↓↓↓ | ↑↑↑ |
| Freund's adjuvant | Depot (+) and immunostimulatory | ↑↑↑ | ↓↓ |
| Oil-in-water | Depot (+++) | ↓ | ↑↑↑ |
| Saponins | Immunostimulatory | ↑↑↑ | ↑ |
| Immune stimulating complexes | Particulate | ↑↑↑ | ↑ |
| Ginsenosides | Immunostimulatory | ↑↑↑ | ↑ |

vaccination needs a fine balance between generating effective immunity and causing damage through an excessive inflammatory reaction.

Pig vaccines based on live attenuated microorganisms (especially viruses) will infect cells and multiply in the body. This pathogenic mechanism triggers a Th1 immune response characterised by generation of cytotoxic T cells (CD8+) that can destroy the cells infected by the virus. A humoral response is also generated (Fig. 5). In summary, vaccines

It is worth highlighting that the adjuvants in commercial vaccines are often a mixture of depot-type, particulate and/or immunostimulatory adjuvants, and their exact composition is protected under patent and unavailable to the public.

based on live attenuated microorganisms are potent, generate cellular and humoral immune responses, and do not need adjuvants in their formulation. They tend to be economic to produce but can have residual virulence and can therefore cause disease. They also do not always require a booster dose (revaccination).

Inactivated microorganisms act as exogenous antigens and stimulate responses by CD4+ receptors on Th2 cells (Fig. 6). Therefore, in principle, they only induce a humoral response. These vaccines are safe, stable and require adjuvants in their formulation. They also often need a booster dose and are expensive to produce. Another significant feature is that they can cause more problems from anaphylactic reactions than other vaccine types, which will be discussed later.

Vaccines based on microorganism subunits contain only fragments of the microorganism that are obtained by physical and chemical processes or by genetic engineering. They usually induce humoral immunity, but little cellular immunity. Their cost varies depending on how they are produced, and are safe and stable. They usually need potent adjuvants and a booster dose, and some antigens and adjuvants can cause adverse reactions. They also have a narrow immunological margin (only induce a response to specific antigens).

DNA vaccines and live vector vaccines might possibly be commercially available in the near future. These contain the relevant antigens, viral or bacterial, that have been genetically modified. The immune response generated by these vaccines is very similar to the response produced by attenuated live microorganisms (Table 3).

Table 3. Differentiation of the immune response according to the type of vaccine used. More plus signs (+) indicate a stronger response.

| Type of vaccine | Th2 (antibodies) | Th1 (cellular) |
|---|---|---|
| Inactivated | +++ | – |
| Subunits | +++ | – |
| Attenuated | ++ | +++ |
| Live vectors | + | +++ |
| DNA | + | ++++ |

**Figure 5.** Attenuated vaccines trigger a Th1 immune response, characterised by the generation of CD8+ capable of destroying cells infected by the virus. They also trigger a humoral response.

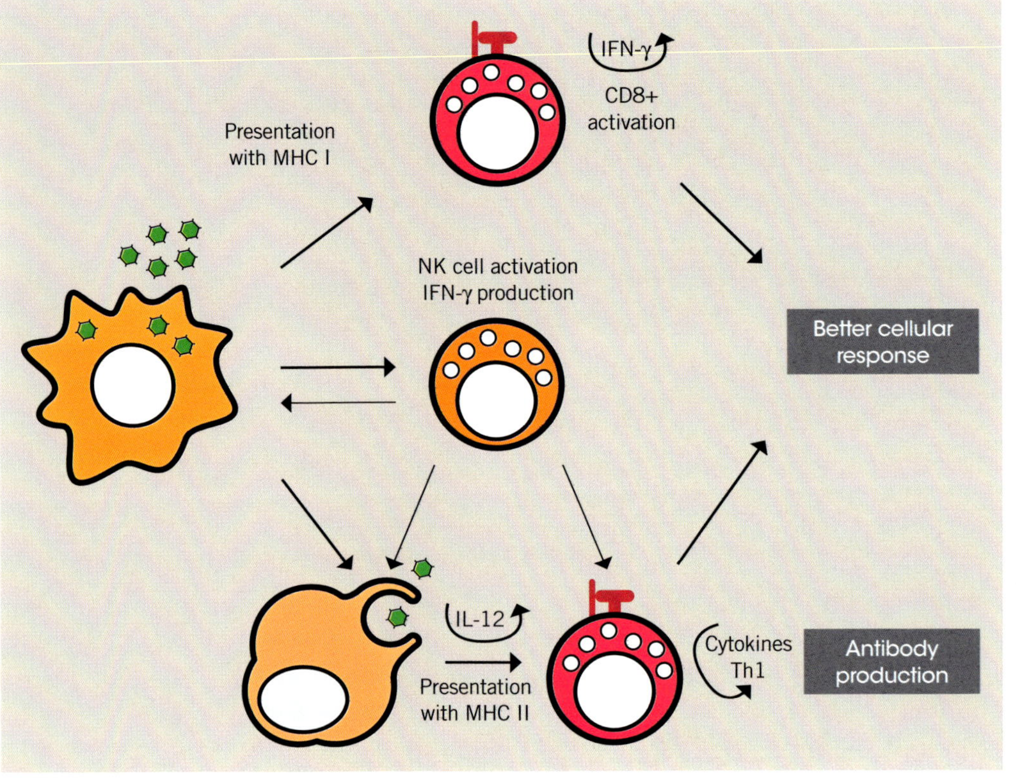


**Figure 6.** The antigens in inactivated vaccines are captured by the APC through endocytosis. The antigen is presented in association with MHC II. The absence of IFN or IL-12 secretion gives rise to Th2 differentiation with preferential production of antibodies.

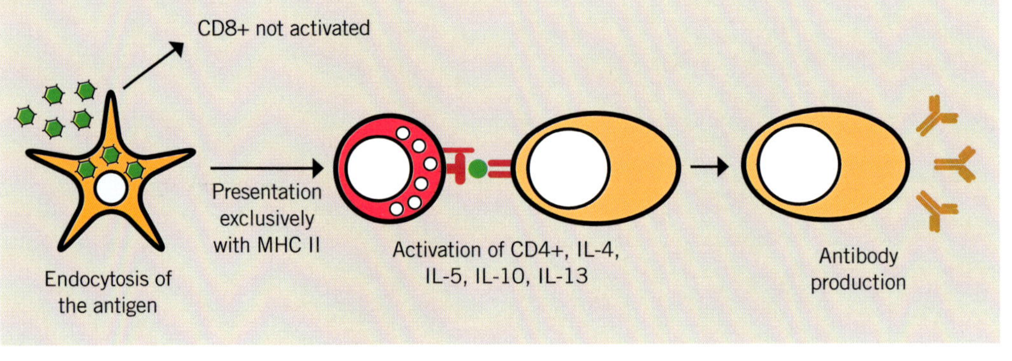

## PRACTICAL VACCINE APPLICATION

The vaccines available for many diseases prevent clinical signs from appearing, but do not prevent infection. Despite this clear limitation, vaccines reduce the morbidity and mortality of many diseases, as they both reduce the probability that the pathogen is transmitted within the population and reduce the effect on individual health by lessening the pathogen damage to various tissues.

> Vaccination has a very positive effect on disease control at a population level.

However, there are also negative aspects of vaccines, such as their cost, accidents or post-administration incidents, and, of significant concern, the potential for vaccine interference with routine diagnostic testing, as many tests are based on detecting antibodies (IgG and/or IgM) in the animal's blood.

The ability to differentiate between the serological response to vaccination and the response to natural infection should be an important objective in vaccine production. A small proportion of the vaccines available do have this feature, and are called marker or DIVA vaccines. However, the vast majority of commercially available vaccines are not marker vaccines. In the case of attenuated vaccines, shedding of microorganisms from the vaccine into the population is an important negative feature.

> Unfortunately, many vaccines do not allow laboratory testing to distinguish vaccinated from infected animals.

The package insert for each vaccine details the dose and the route of administration that should be used. The most common commercial vaccines are administered to pigs by the intramuscular route, but some are suitable for oral, intranasal or intradermal administration. Intramuscular administration requires a clean, sharp needle to minimise damage at the vaccination site. Intradermal administration is of particular interest, as it massively reduces the potential for iatrogenic transmission by using a needle-free device. Intramuscular and intradermal administration generate good systemic immunity, but good mucosal immunity can be much more useful in some diseases. The ideal route of administration in these cases would be oral or intranasal, to generate satisfactory immunity in the digestive or respiratory mucosae respectively. Finally, vaccines are designed to be administered at a particular dose which should never be adjusted to the size of the animal, as vaccines are not designed to use the weight of the individual as a correction factor. Vaccines are designed to contain the correct amount of antigen to trigger a good immune response, and any reduction can result in an inadequate response. From a practical perspective, it may be necessary to generate an adaptive immune response very quickly to a variety of pathogens that can infect the animal, or it may be desirable to minimise animal handling during vaccine administration. In these cases, it is advisable to use vaccines that contain multiple antigens (polyvalent), as using an inappropriate mixture of various separate antigens (and their adjuvants) may fail to generate a good response to one or more of them. Questions have been raised over whether the use of polyvalent vaccines produce a satisfactory immune response, or whether they might increase the likelihood of adverse reactions. Scientific evidence has proven these doubts to be unfounded.

> If the vaccine (the combination of antigens and/or adjuvants) is well designed, it can cause a good immune response to many antigens without increasing the probability of adverse reactions.

The ideal effect of vaccination would be that all animals respond homogeneously, and therefore have a similar level of protection. Figure 7 shows the possible reasons that an individual might not respond to a vaccine as required. The first and most obvious reason that must be ruled out is incorrect administration, whether by an inappropriate route, or because the modified live microorganism was not viable, or because of the persistence of maternal antibodies to this disease in the animal. The package insert for each vaccine must be consulted to prevent maternal antibodies causing vaccine failure. The insert will explain whether there is any interference from maternal immunity and state how many weeks old the piglet will be when this interference ceases to be significant. If there is no information available in this respect (very unlikely), or if autogenous vaccines are used on the farm, it would be very useful to use serological profiles to decide the ideal moment to vaccinate the piglets, as shown in Figure 8. However, vaccine failure can still occur, despite appropriate vaccine administration. This may be because the animal is already infected and does respond to the vaccine, or the vaccine antigen does not provide cross-protection for the pathogen found on the farm (Fig. 7). Another cause of vaccine failure, despite correct administration, is that the animal does not respond because it is immunosuppressed for other reasons (coinfection and/or stress). Additionally, there is biological variation in the population's response to the vaccine.

The precise relationship between the host's genotype and the ability to respond to vaccines is unknown, but it is likely to include major histocompatibility complexes (MHCs) (e.g. the peptides being processed can fail to bind, or bind with a low affinity, to particular receptors) and the host's genes that control cytokine profiles (e.g. in Th1 or Th2 cells). Mutations in these genes could potentially alter the vaccine response.

Adaptive immune responses begin to develop a little time after vaccination, and this period is called the onset of immunity. It is very important to remember this, as the animal is not protected against infection by the pathogen if present in the surroundings during this time. The concept of immunological memory was described in the first chapter, and this consists of the ability to 'remember' an antigen and learn how to destroy it so that the defence system is rapidly activated if the pathogen reappears. The body's ability to develop these specific responses is maintained by the memory cells (B and/or T cells). Another very important parameter is the duration of immunity, which is the period in which adaptive immunity will effectively protect against the pathogen. It is advisable to revaccinate the animals before the end of this period. Finally, the revaccination period depends on whether the vaccine contains live or inactivated organisms, and its route of administration.

A population's immune response always follows a normal distribution curve (Fig. 9). This means that some of the animals develop an inadequate response and are therefore very poorly protected against the pathogen. Others develop a very good immune response and will be extremely well protected and, finally, the vast majority of individuals develop an adequate immune response and will be adequately protected.

**Figure 7.** Reasons why the vaccine might fail to protect the animal (adapted from Tizard, 2013).

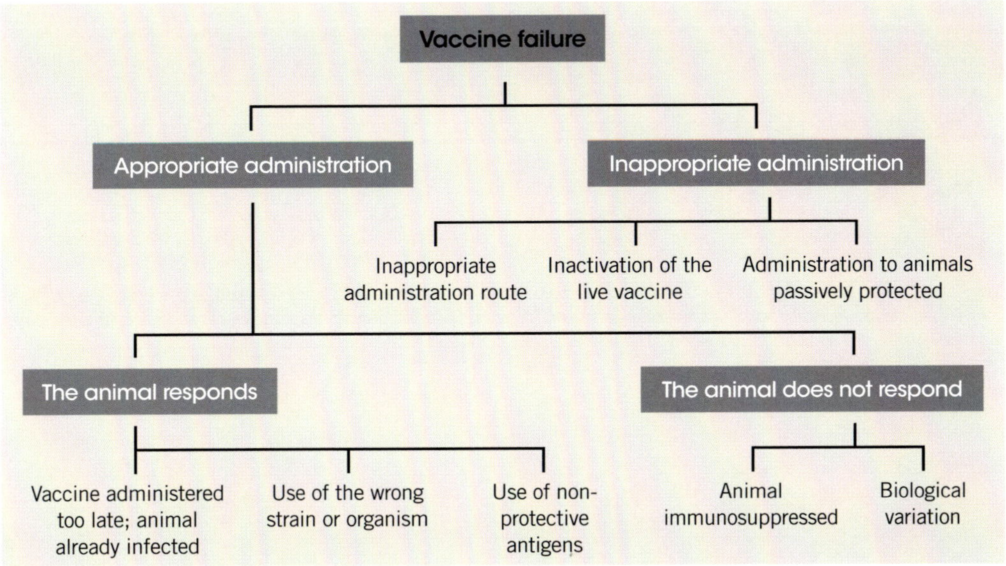

**Figure 8.** Serological profiles of young piglets on a farm.

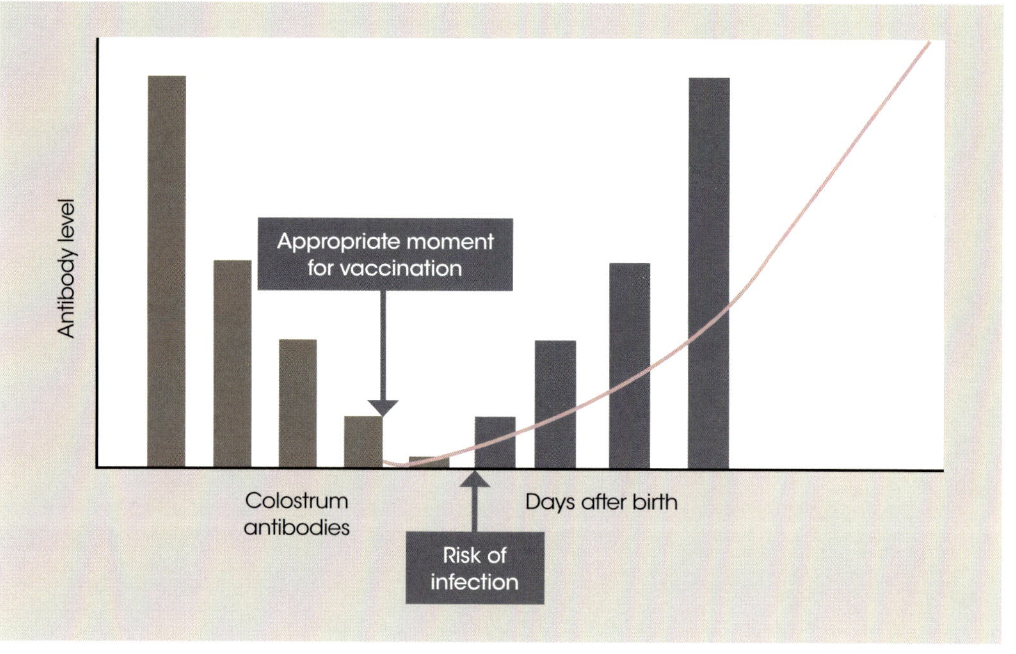


**Figure 9.** Normal distribution of protective immune responses in a population of vaccinated animals. No vaccine can protect 100 % of the population (adapted from Tizard, 2013).

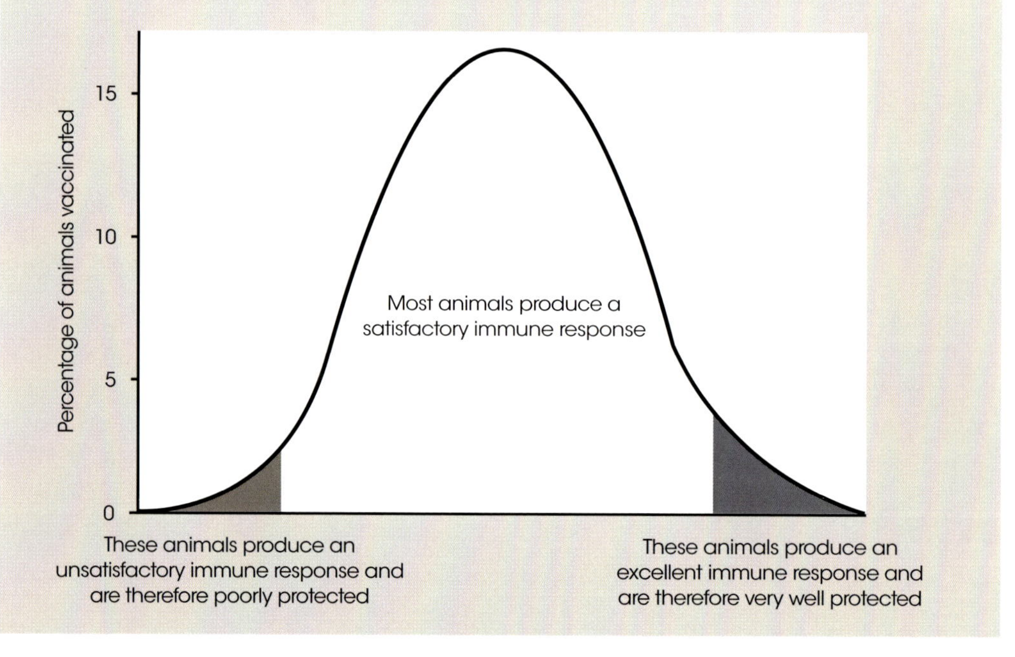

## ADVERSE REACTIONS TO VACCINES

Vaccination is the safest, most reliable and effective method to protect animals against infectious diseases.

> The adverse reactions associated with vaccines are normally temporary and largely consist of inflammation and pain at the vaccination site, and fever and anorexia that tend to abate after a few days.

The inflammatory response at the vaccination site, the starting point for the immune response, may be associated with adverse reactions. These adverse reactions are considered 'normal' and are described in depth in the vaccine package insert, as a requirement of the licensing process. Figure 10 shows all the adverse reactions that can be caused by vaccination. It is important to remember that manufacturing errors are very uncommon, so veterinary surgeons should use licensed vaccines and follow the manufacturer's recommendations for vaccine storage, dose, and usage scrupulously.

These factors should be considered if a decision is taken to use autogenous vaccines, and the veterinary surgeon should demand that the laboratory producing these vaccines adheres to similar quality standards as the pharmaceutical laboratories that specialise in commercial vaccine production. Adverse reactions can be much more severe, and these are shown in Figure 10 as undesirable effects. These responses can be neurological, a foreign body reaction at the vaccination site, or hypersensitivity, which can be type I, III or IV (Fig. 10). Type I hypersensitivity reactions can be seen in pigs and these occur when the individual generates IgE antibodies in responding not only to the immunising antigen but also to other antigens found in the vaccine. These can be antigens from the eggs used to manufacture some viral vaccines, or remains of tissue cultures.

> Creation of vaccines using pathogens isolated from the same farm can be useful under some circumstances, such as when no commercial vaccines are available or when a pathogen displays a wide range of antigenic variation that is not covered by commercial vaccines.

A reaction may be seen in the animal any time from a few minutes to 3 hours after the antigen is administered. Adverse reactions that occur more than 3 hours after administration are not hypersensitivity type I reactions. Another adverse reaction that can occur in pigs is type IV hypersensitivity at the vaccination site. This response is caused by depot–type adjuvants that persist for some time, so it is more common to see this reaction after giving vaccines containing oil-in-water adjuvants than those containing aluminium hydroxide. Table 4 shows adverse reactions after vaccination, their clinical classification and most probable cause. It should be noted that these adverse reactions are so uncommon that it is impossible to demonstrate significant statistical differences in serious adverse reactions between unvaccinated control groups and vaccinated groups.

> These type I hypersensitivity reactions are associated with repeat booster vaccination and are therefore more common with inactivated vaccines.

Figure 10. The main adverse reactions caused by vaccines (adapted from Tizard, 2013).

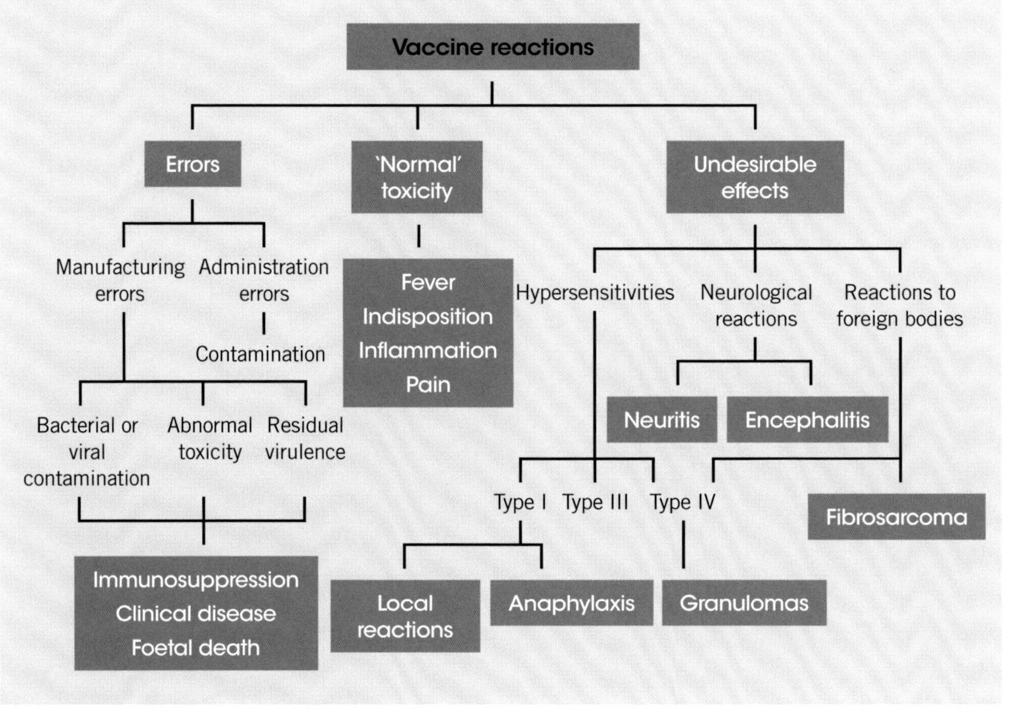

Table 4. Disadvantages of vaccines.

| Type of reaction | | Clinical description | Origin |
|---|---|---|---|
| Generalised reaction | | ■ Hyperthermia<br>■ Anorexia<br>■ Reduced production<br>■ Shock | ■ Pyrogenic effect<br>■ Adjuvant effect<br>■ Stress |
| Allergic reaction | Generalised | ■ Anaphylactic shock<br>■ Delayed reaction | ■ Sensitising factors:<br>■ Heterologous cells<br>■ Serum albumin<br>■ Egg-derived albumin, etc. |
| | Localised | ■ Swelling at the vaccination site | |
| Localised reaction | | ■ Inflammation (pain/necrosis/suppuration) | ■ Oil-based adjuvants<br>■ Type of emulsion<br>■ Inadequate asepsis |
| Various problems | | ■ By a contaminating agent | ■ Contamination of the vaccine<br>■ Faulty manufacture |
| | | ■ Clinical signs of disease | ■ Residual pathogen |
| | | ■ Various diseases | ■ Immunosuppression |

# 03

# TRANSFER OF PASSIVE IMMUNITY TO THE PIGLET

# TRANSFER OF PASSIVE IMMUNITY TO THE PIGLET

## PASSIVE IMMUNITY AND ITS ROLE IN THE PIGLET

### INTRODUCTION

In mammals, maternal immunity is transferred to the progeny through the placenta or by ingesting mammary secretions after birth. The mammary gland is a very specialised tissue that has evolved to feed the newborn offspring. Indeed, milk production after parturition is a characteristic that differentiates mammals from other vertebrates. Serum antibodies are transferred through the placenta in some mammals such as humans, lagomorphs and rodents, but not in pigs, which have placentas separated by three maternal layers of tissues (epitheliochorial) that are impermeable to immunoglobulins. Therefore, piglets are hypo- or a-gammaglobulinaemic at birth.

The porcine foetus begins to develop an immune response from 70 days of gestation, but the newborn piglet's immune system is not completely developed until around four weeks of age. However, the newborn piglet is exposed to many infectious agents after birth (including *Escherichia coli*, transmissible gastroenteritis virus and porcine rotavirus) that can proliferate rapidly before the animal has developed an effective immune response, leading to neonatal disease. Newborn animals are predisposed to these diseases, and this can be explained by the lack of previous antigenic sensitisation that would enable the animal to produce their own immune response quickly enough to provide adequate protection.

### COLOSTRUM, TRANSIENT MILK AND MATURE MILK

The mammary gland in the sow is made up of adipose tissue and a highly organised system of ducts that terminate in the mammary alveoli. In the second half of gestation (days 75–90), the alveoli increase in number and size, and the amount of adipose tissue decreases, giving rise to the development of fully differentiated secretory lobules (day 105) and the alveolar lumen becomes noticeably distended by colostrum (Fig. 1). The rapid acceleration of mammary gland growth (mammogenesis) after day 75 of gestation coincides with an increase in the production of hormones that stimulate mammary development, including oestrogens, relaxin and prolactin. The next phase, lactogenesis, coincides with a reduction in oestradiol, cortisone and progesterone levels in the blood. Prolactin levels start to increase in the last quarter of gestation and continue after farrowing, inducing greater mammary gland development in response to suckling.

Mammary secretion in the sow gradually changes from colostrum to transient milk to mature milk, with most colostrum produced before farrowing, and transient and mature milk produced after. Colostrum can be defined as the mammary secretion consumed by newborn piglets in the first 24 hours after the birth of the first piglet. By 34–36 hours after parturition, the secretion produced to day 10 of lactation is termed transient milk, although the most significant changes are seen at hours 72–96 of lactation. Finally, mature milk is defined as the milk secreted from day 10 of lactation until the end of lactation, and its composition remains virtually the same during this entire period (Table 1).

Most (if not all) colostrum is produced before the birth of the first piglet, so production does not depend on suckling by the piglets. The first component of colostrum, β–lactoglobulin, is produced around day 80 of gestation, but the last week of gestation is very important for colostrum production. Colostrum is considered to be the 'elixir of life' due to its abundance of various components (macronutrients and micronutrients, bioactive molecules like immunoglobulins, growth factors and enzymes) that are important for the newborn piglet's survival. The main differences between sow colostrum and mature milk are in their macronutrient and immunoglobulin concentrations, but levels of many of the components of colostrum also change significantly and rapidly, despite the period of colostrum production being very short. In fact, these levels change nearly every hour. For practical purposes, it is enough to differentiate between the composition of early (0 hours), middle (12 hours after farrowing) and late (24 hours after farrowing) colostrum (Table 1). The protein fraction in colostrum provides energy, but also serves other purposes, including the transference of immunity (immunoglobulins) and the stimulation of growth (growth factors). The most significant changes in the protein fraction occur gradually from early to late colostrum. In terms of overall nutritional value, including energy, late colostrum and transient milk are superior to early colostrum due to their higher levels of fat and lactose. Conversely, the immunological and bioactive properties of early colostrum are much greater than late colostrum. For this reason, colostrum should be ingested as soon as possible after birth to optimise the acquisition of passive immunity by the piglet.

## THE ROLE OF COLOSTRUM IN NEWBORN PIGLET SURVIVAL

Survival of the newborn piglet depends on the ingestion of colostrum in the first hours of life. Colostrum gives the newborn piglet passive immunity which originates from antigenic stimulation of the maternal immune system. Low survival of newborn piglets that have not consumed colostrum is also due to the fact that the piglet's energy reserves are low at birth. Energy from liver glycogen, colostrum and transient milk (in the first few days) helps maintain a constant body temperature and keeps the piglet alive. The newborn piglet requires large amounts of energy for physical activity (locomotion, suckling and competition for teats) and thermoregulation.

Table 1. Colostrum, transient milk and mature milk production in sows. Values with different superscript letters indicate statistically significant differences ($p < 0.05$) (Theil et al., 2014).

| | | Colostrum | | | Transient milk | | Mature milk |
|---|---|---|---|---|---|---|---|
| Time postpartum | | Early (0 h) | Middle (12 h) | Late (24 h) | 36 h | 72 h | Day 17 |
| Chemical composition (g/100 g) | Fat | $5.1^{c}$ | $5.3^{c}$ | $6.9^{bc}$ | $9.1^{a}$ | $9.8^{a}$ | $8.2^{b}$ |
| | Protein | $17.7^{a}$ | $12.2^{b}$ | $8.6^{c}$ | $7.3^{cd}$ | $6.1^{d}$ | $4.7^{e}$ |
| | Lactose | $3.5^{d}$ | $4.0^{c}$ | $4.4^{bc}$ | $4.6^{b}$ | $4.8^{ab}$ | $5.1^{a}$ |
| | Dry matter | $27.3^{a}$ | $22.4^{b}$ | $20.6^{b}$ | $21.4^{b}$ | $21.2^{b}$ | $18.9^{c}$ |
| Energy (kJ/100 g) | | $260^{d}$ | $276^{d}$ | $346^{c}$ | $435^{ab}$ | $468^{a}$ | $409^{b}$ |

| | Early colostrum | Mature milk |
|---|---|---|
| IgG (total) (mg/ml) | 61.8 | 1.6 |
| IgA (mg/ml) | 11.3 | 4.1 |
| IgM (mg/ml) | 3.8 | 1.5 |

Glycogen stores provide enough energy for some 16 hours postpartum, and the energy provided by colostrum should contribute significantly to piglet survival from 16 hours to 34 hours postpartum, as transient milk is not secreted until approximately 34 hours after birth (Fig. 2). In addition to the role of colostrum in neonatal nutrition and immunity, recent research suggests that it also plays a role in tissue development in the piglet, especially affecting the intestinal epithelium and reproductive tract. Sow colostrum actually contains approximately 1500 ng/ml epidermal growth factor (EGF) which accelerates intestinal growth. These 'lactocrine' effects are mediated, at least partially, by hormones in the colostrum. It is important to remember that there is a significant link between improved reproductive efficiency in sows and satisfactory colostrum consumption as newborn piglets (Fig. 3). These data show that colostrum consumption is critical to the animal's life, both in the short–term (preweaning survival) and the long–term (future reproductive performance).

**Figure 1.** Transfer mechanism for cellular immunity (colostrum) and humoral immunity (colostrum and milk) (Salmon et al., 2009).

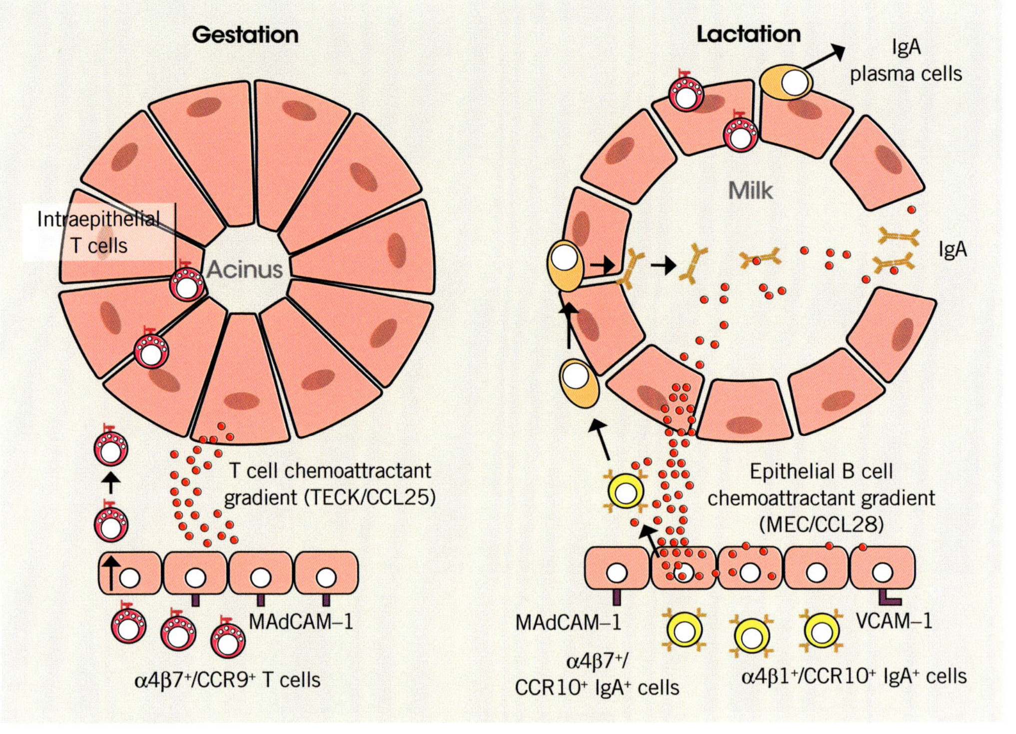


**Figure 2.** Sources of energy for the newborn piglet (Theil et al., 2014).

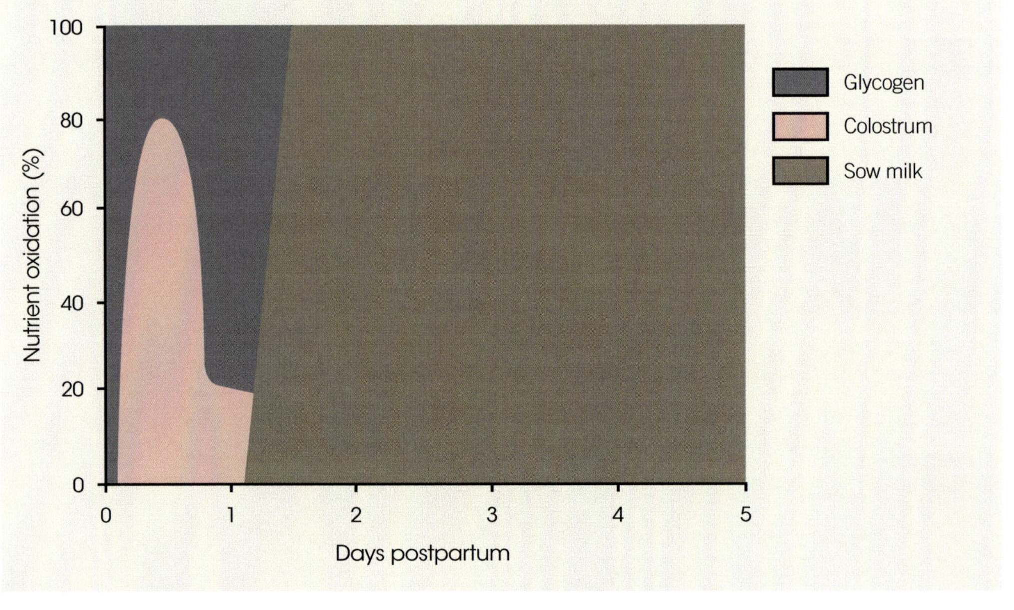

**Figure 3.** Reproductive success of sows as a function of their colostrum consumption as newborn piglets (Vallet et al., 2015).

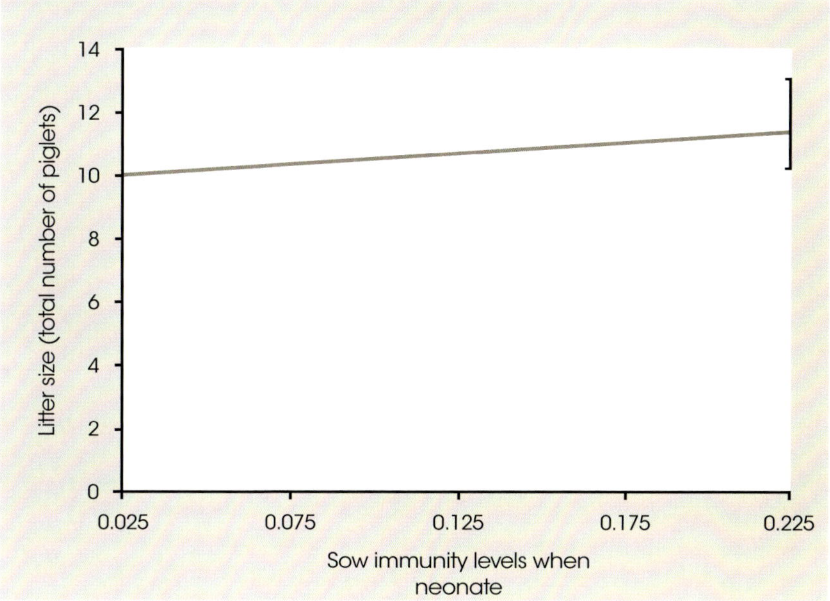


Neonatal mortality is an important cause of preweaning production losses, and the first 24 hours after birth are the most critical, with 28 % of preweaning mortality occurring during this period. Piglets that either consume no colostrum at all, or do not consume enough, will be stunted and therefore more likely to be crushed or to catch infectious diseases. Consuming enough colostrum can reduce the preweaning mortality rate, reducing losses to the production system. Various studies have been carried out to evaluate the amount of colostrum that should be consumed, and mortality has been found to increase significantly in piglets that consumed <200 grams. In one study, the actual mortality rate was around 10 % in piglets that consumed >200 g, 34 % in those ingesting 100–200 g, and 63 % in piglets consuming <100 g. Thus an intake of 200 g colostrum/piglet or 180 g/kg weight at birth seems to be the minimum required to minimise the risk of mortality. Other authors have obtained similar results in terms of mortality (Fig. 4). These mortality results are also linked to the piglets' potential productivity, and an average consumption of 250 g colostrum/piglet is recommended for good body weight gain (Fig. 5) and to reduce the probability of poor productivity at 42 days of age (Fig. 6).

**Figure 4.** Probability of piglet death at 42 days old as a function of colostrum consumption and birth weight (Ferrari et al., 2014).

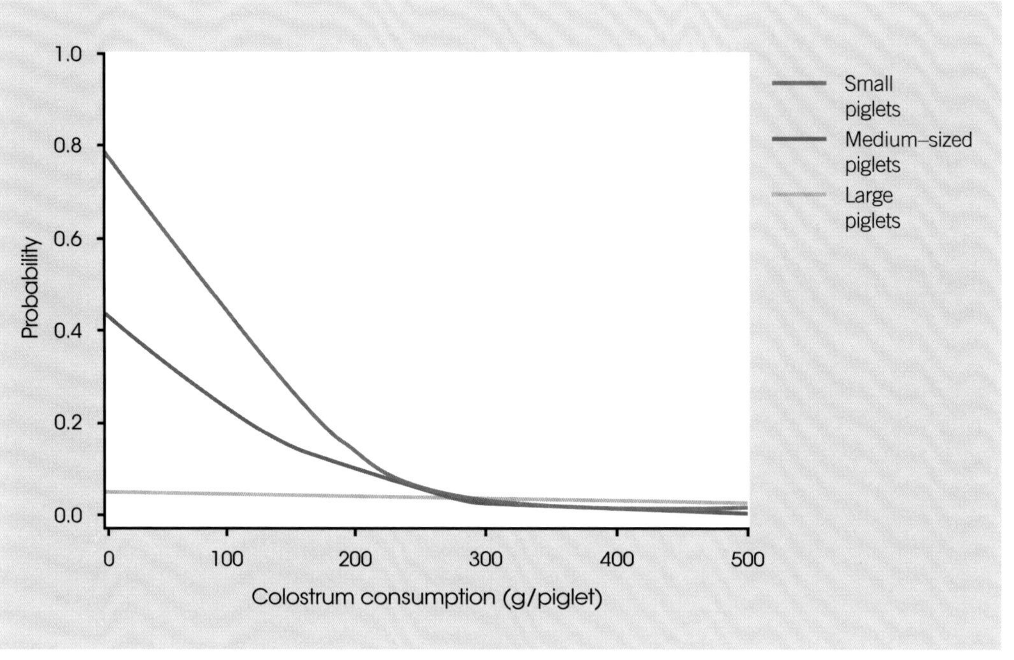


**Figure 5.** Piglet weight at 42 days old as a function of colostrum consumption (Ferrari et al., 2014).

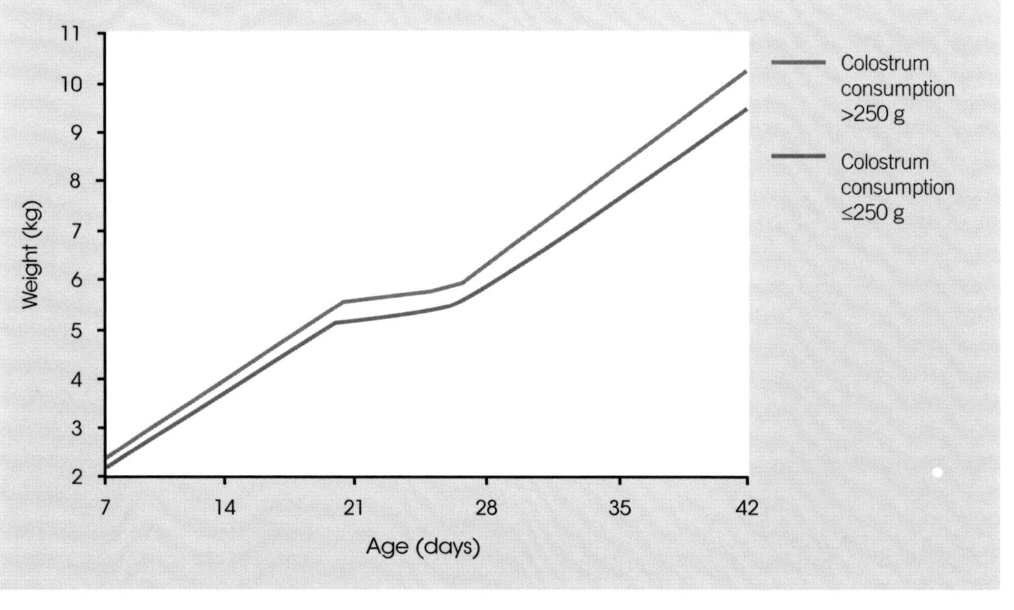

**Figure 6.** Probability of poor productivity at 42 days old as a function of piglet colostrum consumption and birth weight (Ferrari et al., 2014).

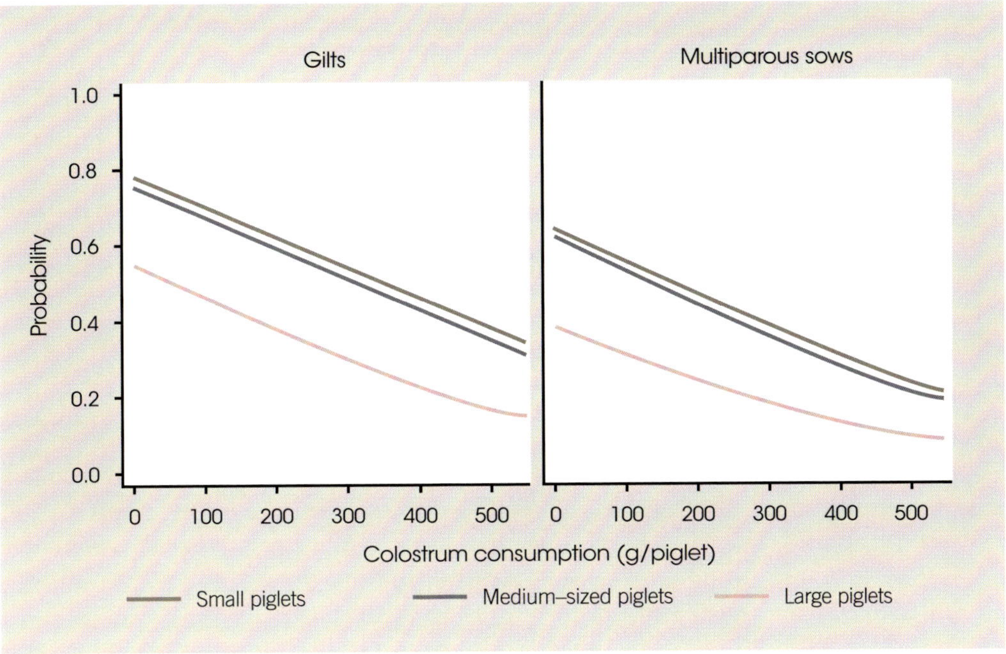


# TRANSFER OF HUMORAL AND CELLULAR IMMUNITY

## INTRODUCTION

Colostrum is an extraordinarily complex mammary secretion that contains lactose, fat and proteins in proportions that change very quickly from birth (early colostrum) until 24 hours postpartum (late colostrum) (Table 1). The importance of lactose and fat in providing energy to the piglet, especially between 16 and 34 hours postpartum has already been mentioned. The proteins in colostrum are also very important for the piglet, as they include immunoglobulins, which are essential elements of humoral acquired immunity. Colostrum also contains many cells; in fact, there are >1 × $10^6$ cells/ml and the piglet is estimated to obtain 5.0–7.0 × $10^8$ maternal cells daily. A relatively large proportion of these are lymphocytes (15–25 %).

Colostrum consumption depends not only on the sow's ability to produce it, but also on the piglet's ability to drink it from the teats. It is worth noting that gilts usually produce colostrum of a poorer quality than multiparous sows, and their piglets (usually smaller) are less able to acquire the colostrum from their mothers (Fig. 7). These two factors cause the level of passive immunity to be lower in piglets born to gilts.

**Figure 7.** Colostrum quality in the first 24 hours postpartum as a function of sow parity (Quesnel, 2011).

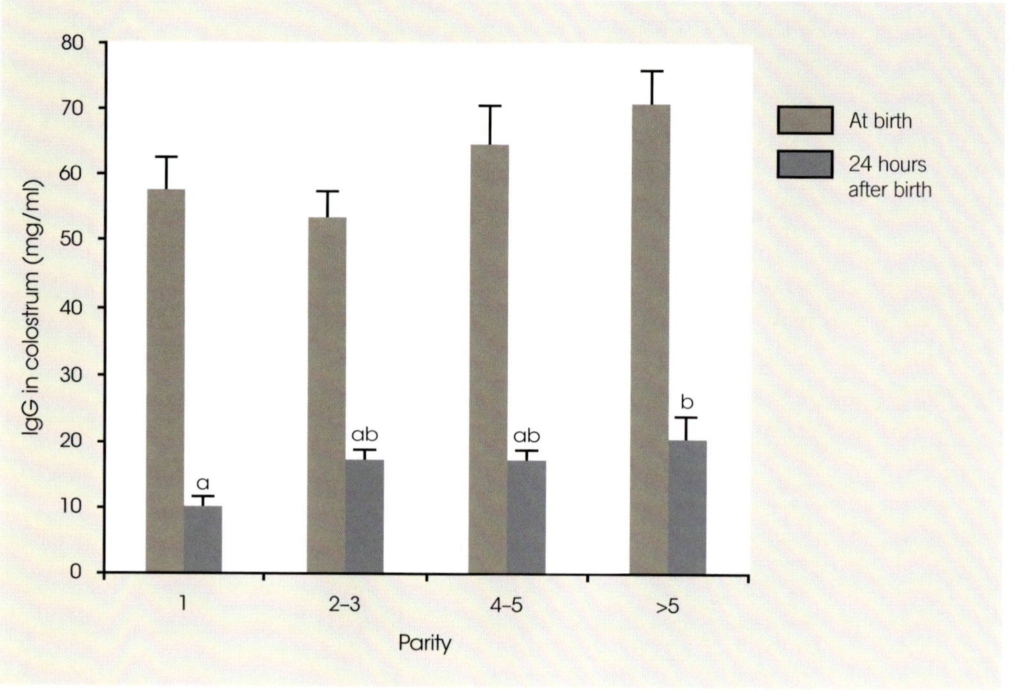


## HUMORAL IMMUNITY

Sow colostrum contains approximately 11 times more immunoglobulins (IgA, IgG and IgM) than mature milk (Table 1), because during colostrum production, immunoglobulins are concentrated in the plasma. Moreover, maternal immunoglobulins are concentrated from the blood to the colostrum in the mammary gland by a mechanism which depends on immunoglobulin receptors (Fig. 1). Scientific studies have demonstrated that almost 100 % of the IgG, 40 % of the IgA and 85 % of the IgM in the colostrum comes from the sow's serum. IgG is the most abundant immunoglobulin in colostrum (81 %), and IgA is the most abundant in the sow's mature milk (57 %). The IgA to IgG ratio varies between 0.61 and 0.22 in colostrum, and 2.1 and 6.96 in mature milk. A very high proportion of IgA is synthesised in the mammary gland. The changes in immunoglobulin levels in mammary secretions reflects the ability of sows to transfer maternal immunity to their progeny.

The immature structure of the neonatal intestine allows immunoglobulins to be absorbed during the first 24–36 hours after birth. Levels of IgG and IgA in the piglet after colostrum has been ingested suggest that absorption of colostrum immunoglobulins is non–selective, as serum levels of IgG and IgA in the piglet follow the ratios of IgG and IgA in the sow's colostrum. Later, the mature intestine does not allow these macromolecules to be absorbed; this phenomenon is called intestinal closure. Therefore, the IgGs ingested in colostrum are absorbed as intact molecules before intestinal closure. As mentioned in the first chapter, IgG is important for functioning of the immune system. After birth, IgG levels in the colostrum decrease rapidly to a low level, while IgA levels only decrease slightly. The IgA ingested in both colostrum and mature milk is important to protect the gastrointestinal tract on a local level and IgA is essential to prevent digestive problems during the neonatal period. This lactogenic immunity is actually widely based, as there is 'communication' between the respiratory, digestive and genitourinary mucosae, so the immune response generated on a local level (basically of humoral and IgA –type) in the respiratory, digestive and genitourinary mucosae appears in the mammary secretions due to migration of IgA–producing B cells through the regional lymphatic ganglia and blood to the mammary gland (Fig. 8).This mechanism is mediated by a molecule (MadCAM–1) expressed in the venules of the Peyer's patches, the intestinal lamina propria and the mammary glands (Fig. 1), and by the a ligand at the lymphocyte level (integrin $\alpha4/\beta7$) that binds to the MadCAM–1 and allows lymphocytes to pass from some compartments to others. The presence of IgA in the milk could be due to selective transport of dimeric IgA from the induction site to the blood, and from the blood by translocation through the mammary epithelium to the milk, or by migration of IgA–producing B cells from the induction site (intestine, and genitourinary and respiratory tracts) to the mammary gland, where it is transformed locally in plasma cells that produce IgA in the milk. IgAs are very important in establishing the intestinal microbiota and preventing food intolerances.

Figure 8. Mucosal immunity and its relationship with lactogenic immunity.

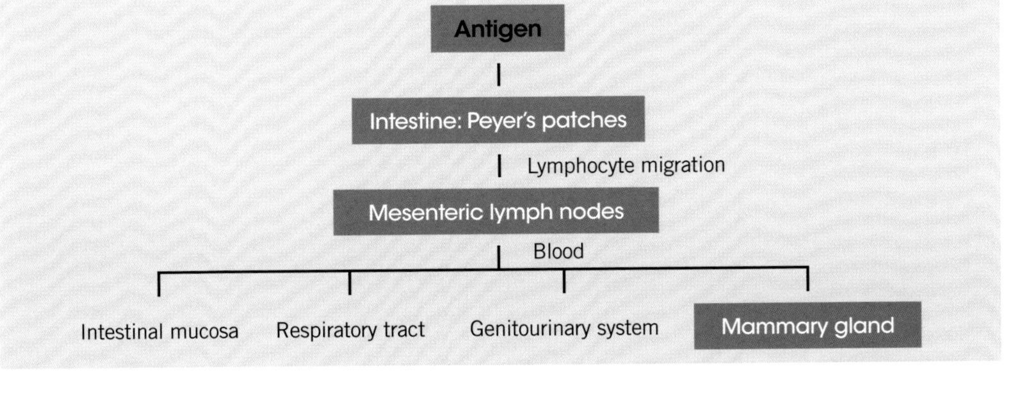

**Figure 9.** Transfer of humoral immunity to *M. hyo* to the piglet. Columns with different superscript letters indicate statistically significant differences ($p < 0.05$) (Bandrick et al., 2014).

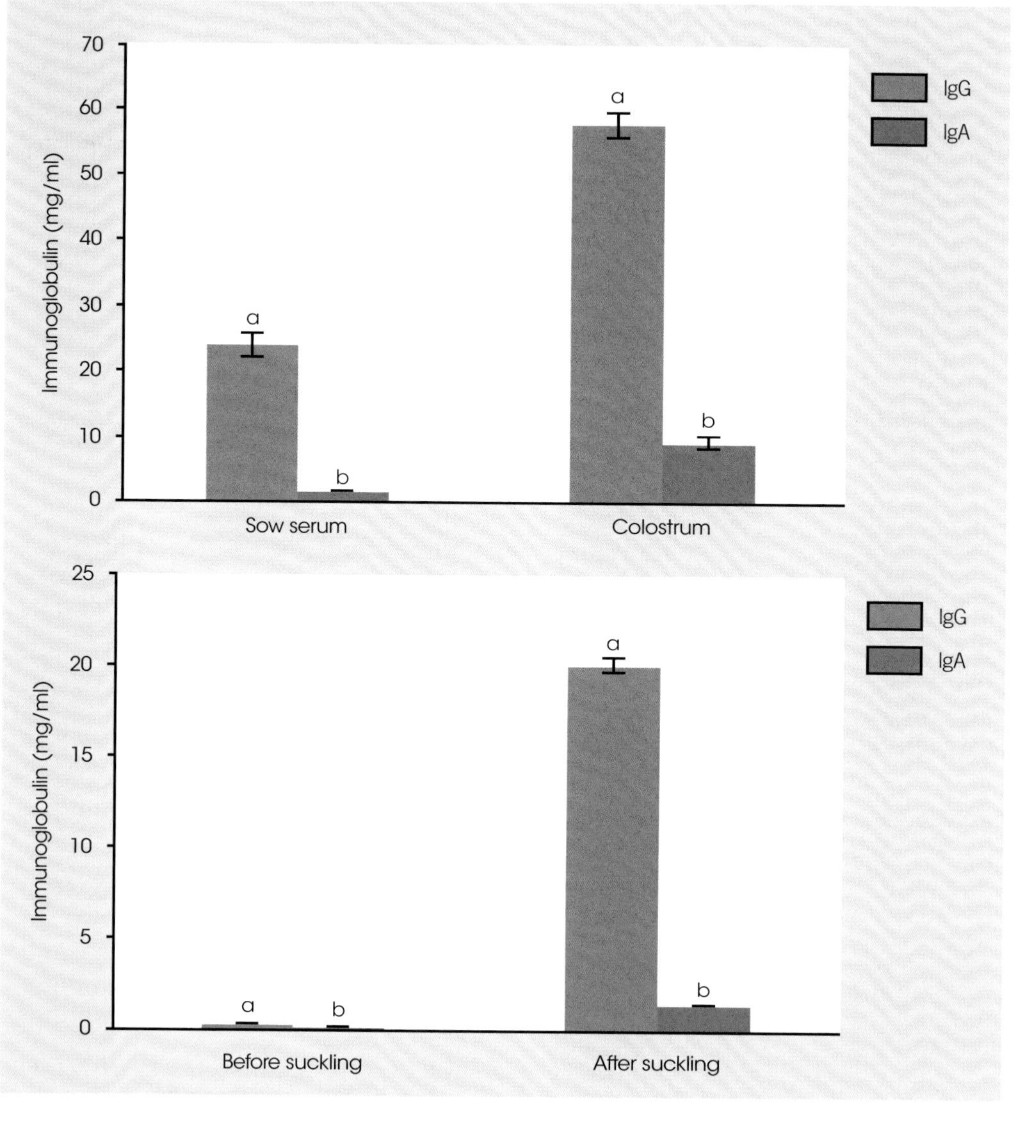


Figure 9 shows data on the transfer of humoral immunity to *Mycoplasma hyopneumoniae* (*M. hyo*) to the piglet. The administration of colostrum is clearly essential to give these animals humoral immunity to the pathogen. Colostrum consumption is also related to IgG levels 24 hours after birth, and remains linked to the piglet's IgG titre at weaning (Fig. 10). In conclusion, sufficient colostrum must be consumed to guarantee the piglet derives a high IgG titre from passive immunity.

**Figure 10.** Transfer of humoral immunity to the piglet during the preweaning period. Importance of colostrum consumption (Devillers et al., 2011).

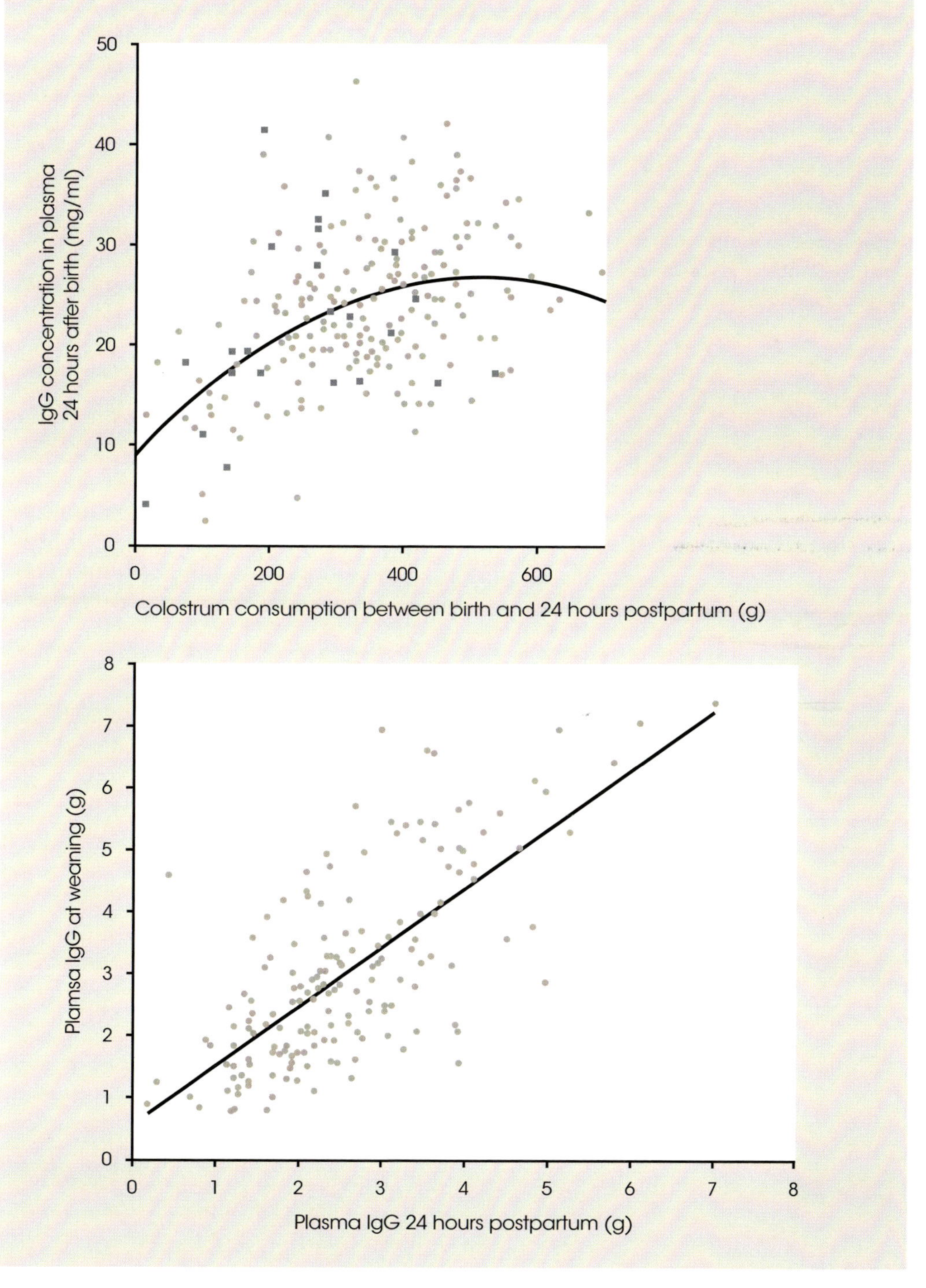

## CELLULAR IMMUNITY

Cell-mediated immunity is very important to the control of many diseases but strangely, the cellular contribution of colostrum has traditionally been disregarded in favour of non-cellular factors, such as immunoglobulins. Mammary secretions of all species contain neutrophils (polymorphs), lymphocytes and macrophages, and approximately $2 \times 10^5$–$10^7$ epithelial cells/ml. The cell types and quantities depend on the stage of development of the mammary gland and other individual factors. For example, colostrum is enriched with phagocytic cells, whereas milk is enriched with epithelial cells. On average, 26 % of the cells found in colostrum are lymphocytes, with B cells being less numerous (≈30 %) than T cells. The T cell subpopulations in colostrum are not representative of those found in the sow's blood (Fig. 11) which suggests that the mononuclear cells in colostrum are selectively concentrated. The percentage of T cells (specifically CD8 and CD4) is significantly lower in the sow's colostrum than in her blood. However, the relative proportions of both subpopulations are very similar in the colostrum and the blood. In pigs, the αβ T cells that express CD4 and CD8 are effector memory cells, and stimulation by their specific antigen induces proliferation of these double-positive (DP) lymphocytes. It is likely that many of the colostrum lymphocytes that are capable of generating an immune response in the piglet are DP effector memory cells. There are also higher levels of γδ T cells in the sow's colostrum than in her blood; in fact, they make up nearly half of the mononuclear cells found in the colostrum. As mentioned in the first chapter, γδ and αβT cells respond to antigens in different ways. γδ T cells are not major histocompatibility complex (MHC)-restricted and they can recognise unprocessed nonprotein antigens. They are also thought to have natural killer (NK) activity and the ability to present antigens. This antigen-presenting cell (APC) aspect is beneficial to the newborn, as neonatal APCs are immature and need greater stimulation to function in a similar way to those of a mature animal. The ability of γδ T cells to evade destruction by the piglet's innate and adaptive immune responses allows it to complement the newborn's own immune system. This advantage can be seen clearly when NK cell activity in piglets that have consumed colostrum is compared to that of the piglet before colostrum is consumed (Fig. 12). Unfortunately, it is not known how maternal lymphocytes are transported across the neonatal intestinal epithelium, but there is evidence to suggest that there is selective lymphocyte transfer. If this is the case, there would be more selective absorption of γδ. The transfer process is mediated by receptors that may be linked to phenotypic cellular changes produced within the colostrum.

It is worth noting that the process of cellular absorption is restricted to colostral cells from the piglet's own mother and it does not occur with colostral cells that have been heat treated or that have come from another sow. In contrast, unlike these immune cells, colostral immunoglobulins cross the neonatal intestinal epithelium and enter the circulation independently of where they came from, so they can be immunoglobulins from another

**Figure 11.** T cell distribution in (a) sow blood and colostrum and (b) piglet blood before and after colostrum ingestion. The mononuclear cells were isolated from sow blood or colostrum, phenotyped with anti-TCR γδ, CD8 or CD4 monoclonal antibodies specific to pigs (n = 16), and analysed by flow cytometry. (a) Levels of T cell subsets in sow blood and colostrum (n = 16). (b) Levels of T cell subsets in piglet blood before colostrum ingestion (before suckling) and again after 24 hours (after suckling) (n = 34). Samples labelled with the same letter are statistically significant: "a" ($p = 0.001$); "b" ($p = 0.0001$) (Bandrick et al., 2014).

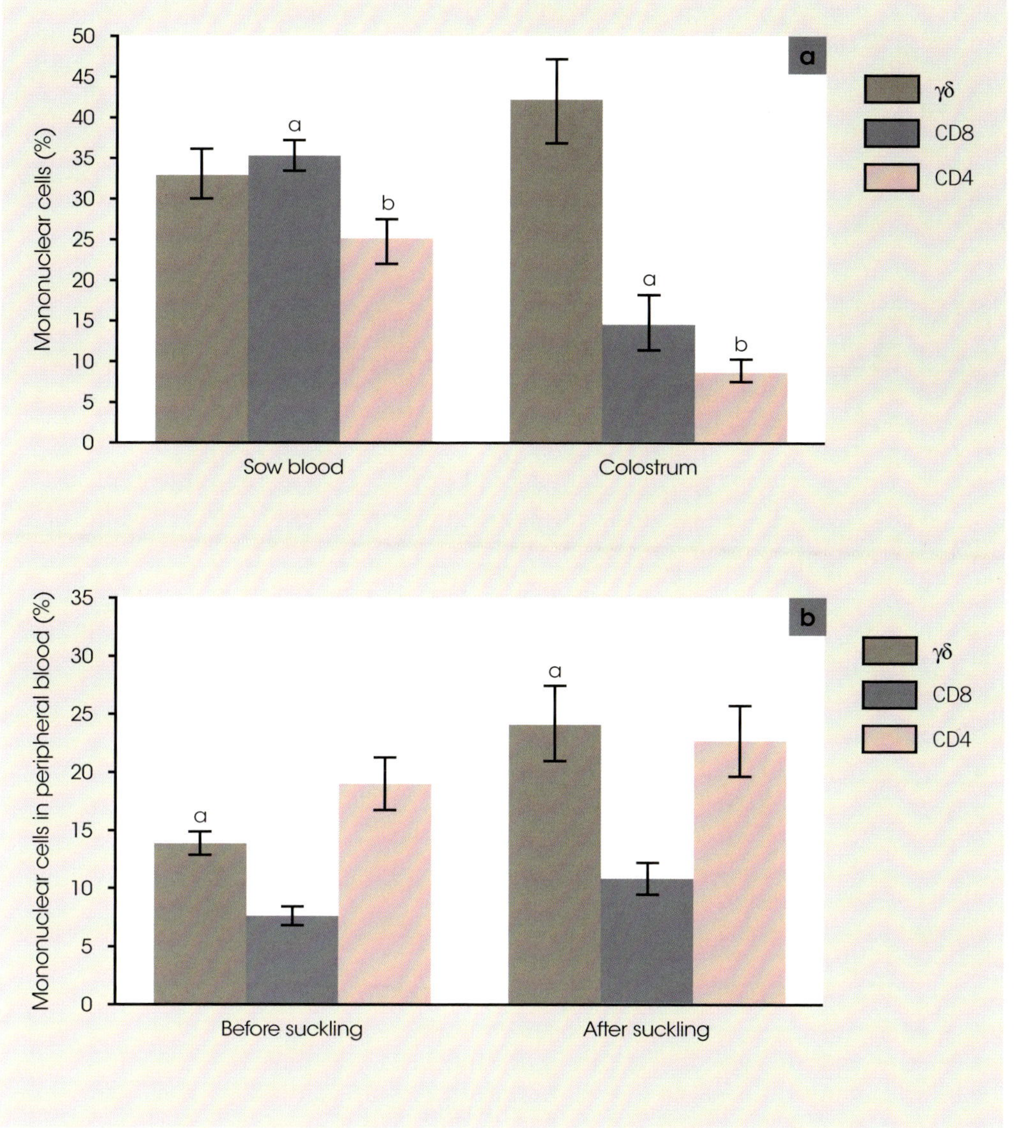

**Figure 12.** NK activity of peripheral and colostral mononuclear cells. NK cell activity was used to assess the functional capacity of the mononuclear cells in sow colostrum (CMC), and sow and piglet blood (PBMC) before and after colostrum consumption. Samples labelled with the same letter are statistically significant ($p < 0.05$) (Bandrick et al., 2014).

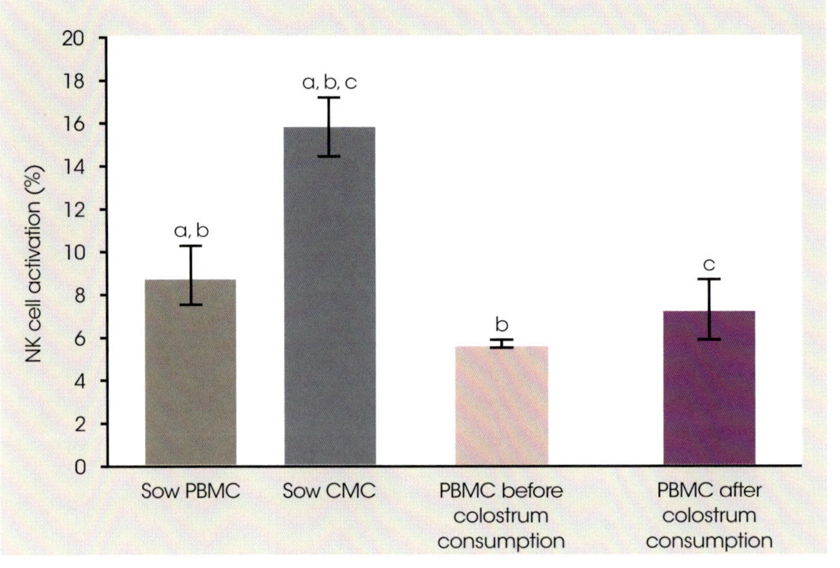


sow or even from another species. The mechanism behind the selective transfer of lymphoid cells in the neonatal intestinal epithelium is still unknown. After crossing the neonatal intestinal epithelium, lymphoid cells are transported to the mesenteric lymph nodes and other tissues. Classic immunological tests (e.g. immune response to a nonspecific mitogen) have demonstrated that these lymphocytes are functional. The high levels of IgG-secreting cells in the piglet's spleen, peripheral lymph nodes and bone marrow at one week of age could also be cells derived from colostral B cells that crossed the intestinal wall.

Figure 13 illustrates the transfer of cellular immunity to *M. hyo* to the piglet. The administration of colostrum was obviously essential to give these animals cellular immunity to this pathogen. So, to conclude, good colostrum consumption by the piglet is essential for good cellular passive immunity.

## STRATEGY FOR IMPROVING THE TRANSFER OF PASSIVE IMMUNITY

Increasing the transfer of humoral and cellular passive immunity from the sow to the piglet is a very important objective that can be achieved by the following measures:

### Vaccination of sows during gestation

Preventive medicine programmes usually involve the vaccination of gestating sows to induce a secondary or tertiary immune response and significantly increase humoral and cellular

**Figure 13.** Transfer of (a) humoral and (b) cellular immunity to *M. hyo*, measured in piglet blood before (n = 7/group) and 24 hours after (n = 10/group) colostrum consumption. The grey columns represent piglets born to vaccinated sows, and the brown columns piglets born to non-vaccinated sows. The error bars correspond to the standard error of the mean; *$p < 0.05$. (a) *M. hyo* antibodies are quantified by the S/P (sample to positive) ratio in piglet serum before suckling and 24 hours after suckling. (b) Specific cellular immunity to *M. hyo* is measured in piglet blood by lymphoproliferation. Antigen-specific lymphoproliferation is determined by subtracting the percentage of non-stimulated lymphoproliferation (mean) from the percentage of lymphoproliferation specific to *M. hyo* (Bandrick et al., 2014).

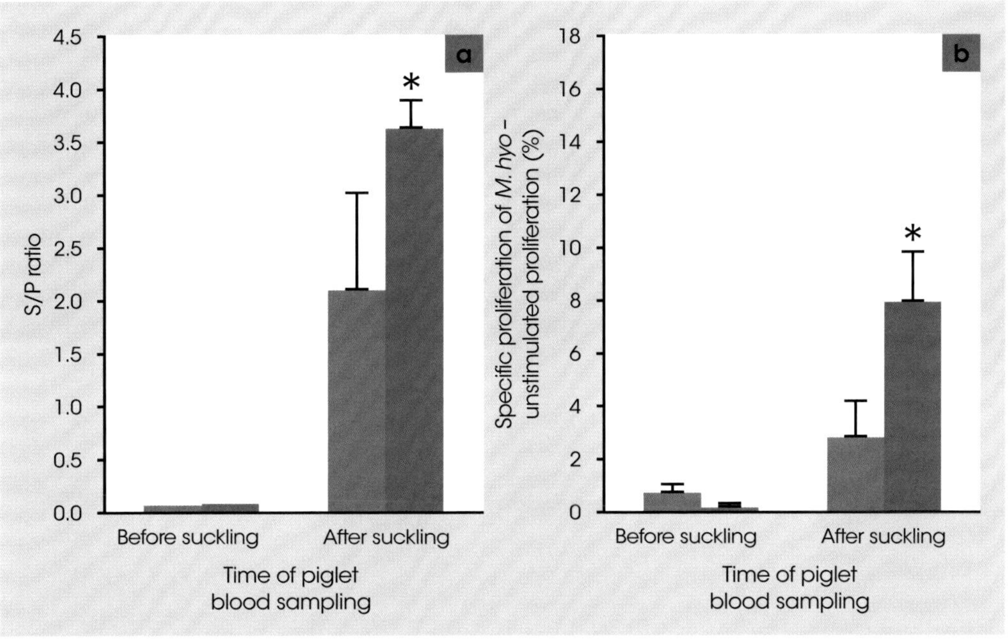


immune response to the targeted pathogen(s). In this way, higher levels of antibodies and cellular immunity can be transferred to the piglet in the colostrum. Figure 14 compares the humoral and cellular immunity acquired by piglets born to sows vaccinated twice against *M. hyo* during gestation, and those born to non-vaccinated sows. Colostral antibody titres were clearly significantly higher in the vaccinated sows, and their piglets also acquired a better cellular immune response to the pathogen. The sows must be vaccinated correctly, and the vaccine must also be capable of generating the type of response required (helper T cells type Th1 or Th2) depending on the pathogen against which protection is required. The chapter that follows will discuss the most important porcine diseases where sows are vaccinated as an important part of a preventive medicine programme.

## Ingestion of sufficient colostrum

The importance of colostrum consumption for piglet survival in the preweaning period has already been discussed. It is essential to optimise the colostrum consumed by each piglet, and this point will be developed in the final chapter of the book.

**Figure 14.** Vaccinating sows against *M. hyo* as a strategy to increase the transfer of (a) humoral and (b) cellular immunity. Samples with different letters indicate statistically significant differences ($p < 0.05$) (Bandrick et al., 2014).

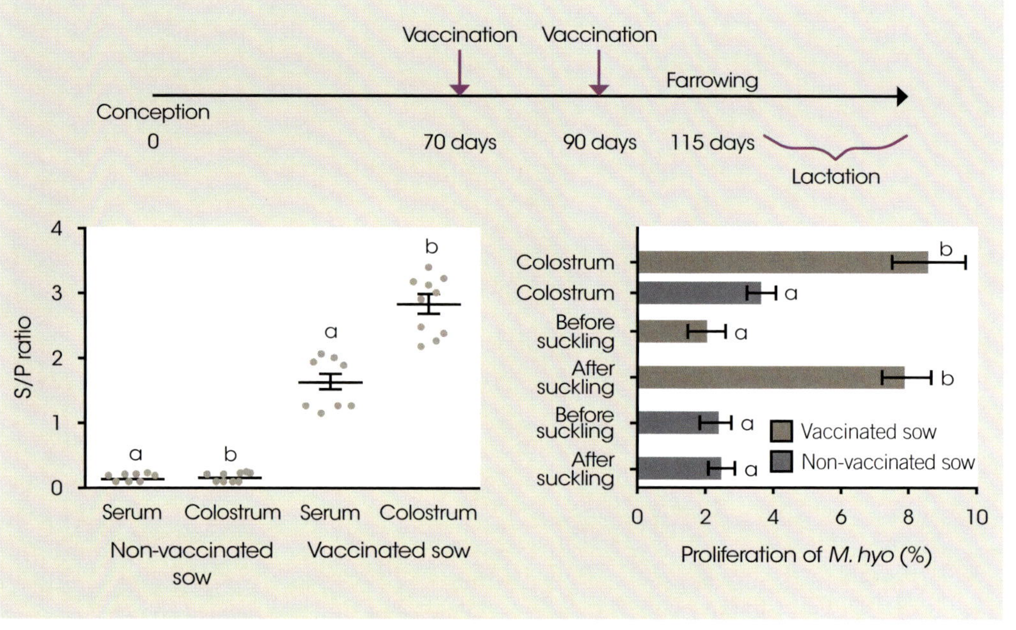


## INTERFERENCE WITH ACTIVE IMMUNITY BY PASSIVE IMMUNITY

### INTRODUCTION

It is very common to vaccinate piglets during the first 3 weeks of life as part of a preventive medicine programme and there are many vaccines that can be administered to piglets during this preweaning stage, following the recommendations issued by the pharmaceutical manufacturers. Vaccination of newborn and suckling piglets is problematic for two reasons: the immune system is immature in the newborn piglet, and the animal has taken in both humoral and cellular immunity through the colostrum.

The neonatal immune system differs significantly from that of adult animals: newborns have fewer APCs, lower levels of costimulatory molecules and less surface expression of MHC II. They also have a lower capacity to produce cytokines (particularly IL-12) in response to stimulation of the Toll-like receptors (TLR). CD4 T cells also show a natural bias towards a Th2 response rather than a Th1 response, so it is likely that the neonatal immune system will respond more effectively with a humoral adaptive immune response rather than a cellular one. Newborns also possess a relative abundance of regulatory T cells (natural immunosuppressants). These cells secrete large amounts of interleukin-10 (IL-10) and transforming growth factor beta

(TGF-β), which promote tolerance-inducing APCs and suppress the effector T cell response, the effects of which include defective plasma cell differentiation. In summary, newborns respond to the immune challenge with an adaptive humoral response which is both qualitatively and quantitatively weaker than the immunologically mature animal. Looking at these differences in the immune response between newborns and adult animals suggests that neonatal immunity is closely regulated, and aims to encourage microbial colonisation and prevent adverse proinflammatory responses. Unfortunately, this also causes vulnerability to infection during the early stages of life. Finally, some other components of colostrum also have an important effect on the neonatal immune response. The corticosteroids in colostrum are immunosuppressant, and the cytokines include proinflammatory factors (TNF-α, IL-1β and IL-6), anti-inflammatory factors (TGF-β and IL-10), growth promoters (erythropoietin, granulocyte colony stimulating factor and macrophage colony stimulating factor [IL-8 / CXCL8 and CCL5]), and agents that promote a Th1-type response (interferon [IFN]-γ and IL-12) and a Th2 response (IL-6, IL-4 and IL-10). However, the predominant lactogenic cytokines (TGF-β1 and IL-4) are involved in strengthening the Th2-type response and reducing the immune response in newborns.

The neonatal immune system is too immature to generate a comparable immune response to that found in adult animals. These are other ways in which the humoral and cellular immunity acquired from colostrum ingestion can modify the immune responses in newborns.

## INTERFERENCE WITH THE DEVELOPMENT OF HUMORAL IMMUNITY

Maternal immunisation is commonly used in veterinary medicine, strengthening passive immunity by increasing the transfer of antibodies from the mother to the piglets. In current production systems, sows are routinely vaccinated against a series of bacterial and viral pathogens. These vaccines induce production of high levels of IgG, IgM and IgA antibodies that are transferred passively to the piglet, increasing the duration of both systemic (Fig. 15) and mucosal (Fig. 16) immune protection against neonatal infections. These passively acquired antibodies enter the bloodstream in the newborn piglet and act as a 'protective shield' throughout the whole body in the same way as actively produced antibodies. However, there are significant differences in the action of passively transferred IgG and IgA antibodies. IgG antibodies are present in the newborn's bloodstream in small quantities that decline with time, and they are responsible for suppressing the active immune responses that vaccines aim to generate. Conversely, IgA antibodies are supplied continuously in the mother's milk and protect the gastrointestinal tract against pathogens without having any effect on the active immune response.

In all mammalian species, maternal antibodies significantly reduce or eliminate antibody production following vaccination of the newborn progeny. It is worth noting that this effect is to be observed using common vaccines (live attenuated, inactivated and subunit vaccine). This effect should be considered, because the reduction or absence

Figure 15. Dynamics of (a) IgG and (b) IgA antibodies to a model antigen (with which the sow was vaccinated) in the serum during the first 28 days of life in the piglet (Netchvatalova et al., 2011).

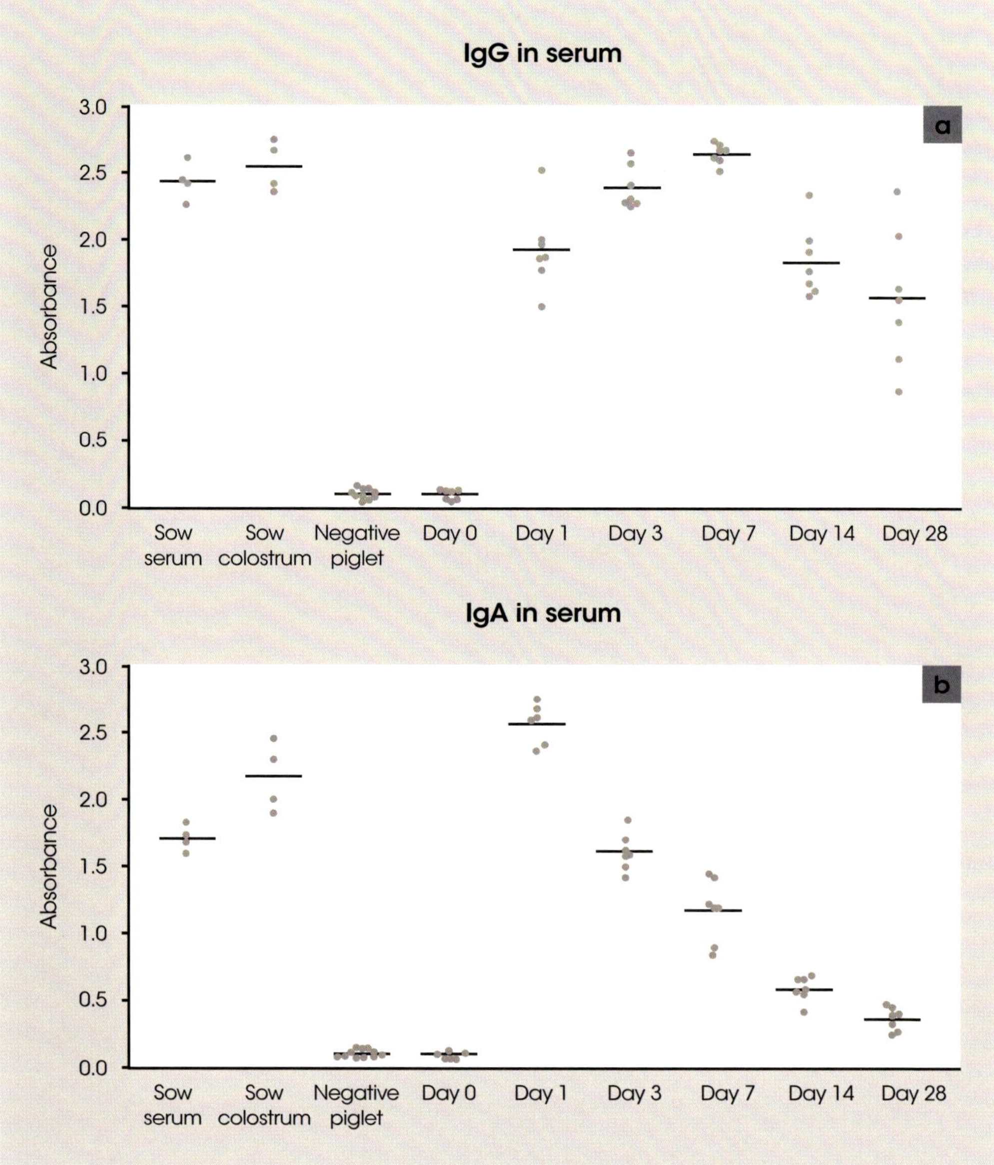

Figure 16. Dynamics of (a) IgG and (b) IgA antibodies to a model antigen (with which the sow was vaccinated) in bronchoalveolar lavage during the first 28 days of life in the piglet (Netchvatalova et al., 2011).

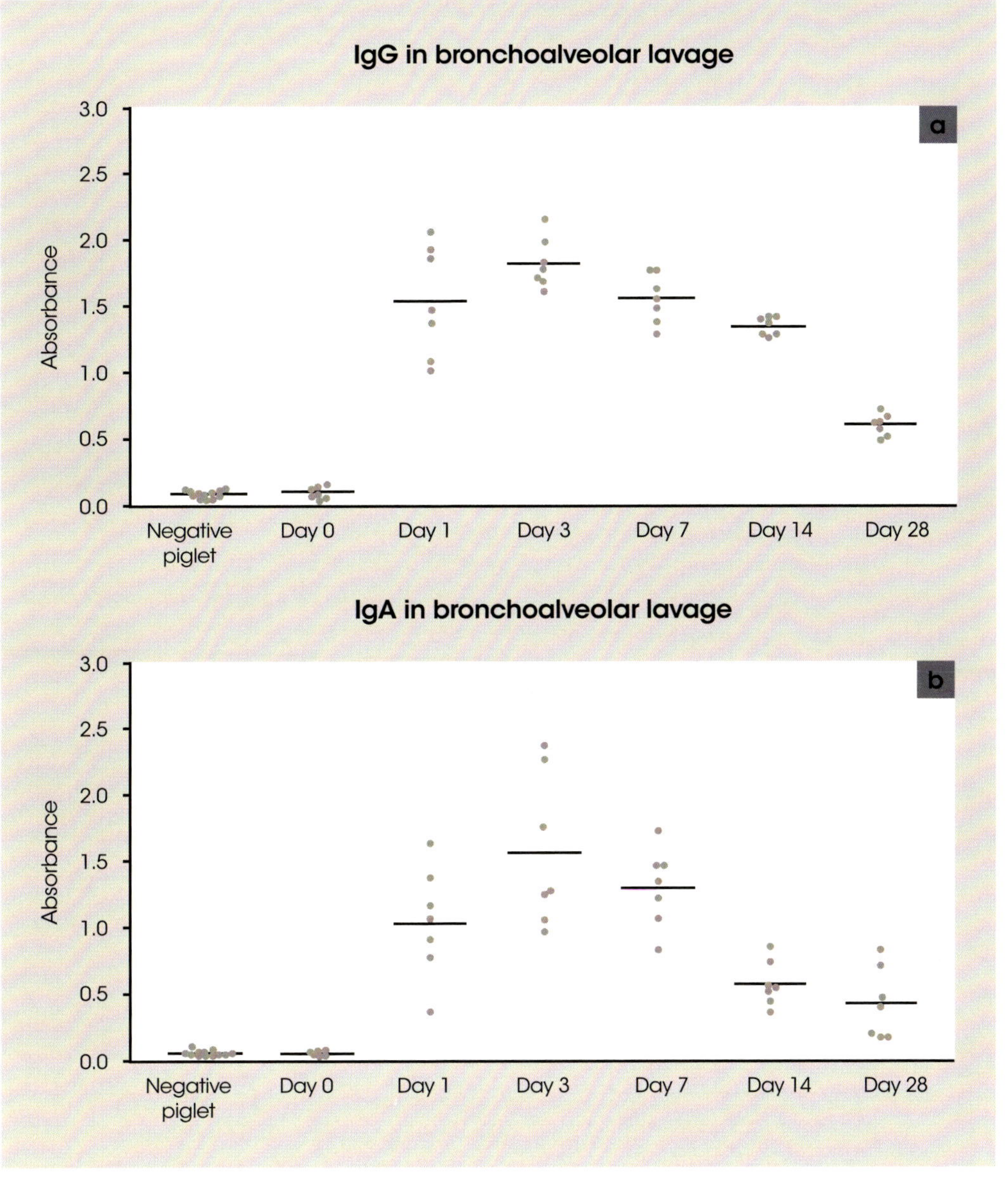

of antibodies can reduce or eliminate protection against the disease. The degree of the blocking effect of maternal antibodies is related to the amount of antibodies present in the newborn after colostrum consumption, so the highest antibody titres persist for longer, as their half-life is constant, although this is determined by the rate that the antibodies acquired through the colostrum are metabolised. Ultimately, maternal antibody titres decrease because the antibodies are metabolised and thus no longer offer protection. However, in both humans and animals, even titres of maternal antibody that are too low to be protective can still inhibit the response to vaccination against infectious diseases. The antibody level at the moment of vaccination crucially affects the humoral immune response in young piglets. This effect could be seen when porcine circovirus type 2 (PCV2) vaccines was administered to piglets with titres of maternal antibodies to this virus (Fig. 17). Animals with maternal antibody titres of 8 (using the immunoperoxidase monolayer assay technique [IPMA]) showed neither an increase nor a decrease in their levels of antibodies following vaccination against PCV2. However, levels in animals with titres of 4 showed an increase, and levels in animals with titres of over 10 a decrease in antibodies, following vaccination. In the case of Aujeszky's disease, various studies have demonstrated that vaccinating against this virus with live attenuated vaccines induced specific immune responses in newborn piglets, including in the presence of maternal antibodies. However, the size of the response depended on the amount of antibodies present at the moment of vaccination, thus demonstrating the existence of interference from maternal antibodies to Aujeszky's disease virus. Clearly, these antibodies hinder optimum protection from vaccination.

This interference with the development of humoral immunity when maternal antibodies are present involves a series of possible mechanisms, including some that neutralise live attenuated vaccines and others that involve feedback on antibody production.

## Neutralisation of attenuated live vaccines

Maternal antibodies can neutralise an attenuated vaccine virus, which needs to reproduce itself to generate an immune response. This effect reduces the amount of viral antigen below a certain (undefined) threshold and interferes with the development of satisfactory immune recognition. Maternal antibodies not only suppress replication in live attenuated vaccines, but also in subunit vaccines and vector vaccines. Non-neutralising antibodies also interfere with the development of immunity generated by live attenuated vaccines.

## Antibody feedback mechanism

Regulation of antibody feedback is a phenomenon where injecting an antigen and a monoclonal antibody specific to that antigen at the same time reduces or inhibits the generation of antibodies specific to that antigen. This suppression increases with the quantity and affinity of the particular antibody and is independent of the immunoglobulin isotype. This phenomenon can be explained by two principal mechanisms: masking of the epitope and B cell regulation by a receptor called Fcγ IIB (FcγRIIB).

**Figure 17.** Increase in PCV2 antibody titre in piglets 21 days after vaccination according to the antibody titre at the moment of vaccination (3 weeks of age) (Fraile et al., 2012).

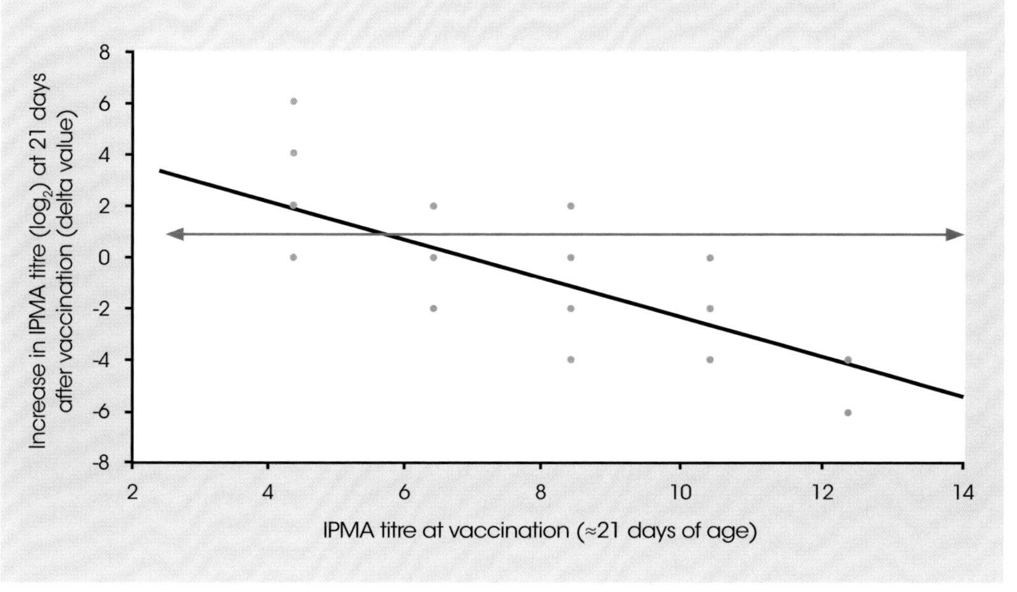


## B-cell epitope masking

This theory states that antibodies can cover critical epitopes and hide them from recognition by B cells if there is enough antibody. Initially, it was thought that all the epitopes on an antigen needed to be covered by antibodies to inhibit recognition by B cells (epitope-specific suppression). However, it has been demonstrated that a monoclonal antibody to an epitope can suppress B cell recognition of the entire antigen (non-epitope–specific suppression). Even low levels of antibodies are known to be able to inhibit antibody production, and the role of epitope masking in suppressing antibody production has always been the subject of debate.

## Inhibition of B-cell activation by signals mediated by the Fc receptor

B cells express the FcγRIIB receptor on their surface, and this can bind to maternal antibodies (Fig. 18). This receptor is in close proximity to the B-cell receptor (BCR), and it has been demonstrated in vitro that in this region, the IgG specific to the BCR binds to the BCR through the antigen-binding site in the variable domain and to the FcγRIIB receptor at the constant domain of this shared region. This proximity inhibits activation of the B cells specific to the antigen. This mechanism has been demonstrated in genetically modified mice that do not have FcγRI, FcγRIIB or FcγRIII. These animals have a stronger acquired humoral response than animals that are not genetically modified, which suggests the absence of a feedback mechanism to regulate B cell responses and antibody titres.

**Figure 18.** Blocking mechanism hindering development of humoral immunity in the presence of maternal antibodies.

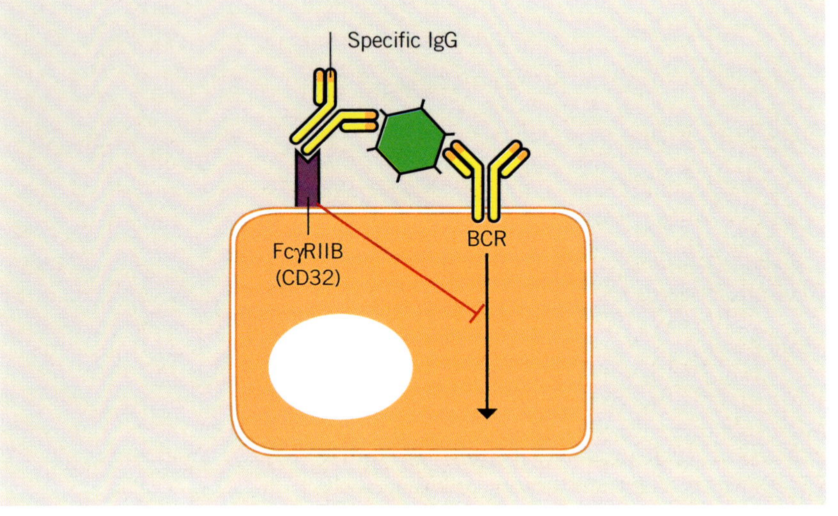


## INTERFERENCE WITH THE DEVELOPMENT OF CELLULAR IMMUNITY

The immaturity of the neonatal immune system has already been described, and this is clearly apparent in the adaptive cellular immune response. The acquisition of a passive adaptive cellular immune response seems to be important for the newborn to face various challenges, and may have a significant effect on the outcome of certain types of infection. However, maternal humoral and cellular immunity seems to interfere with the newborn's ability to develop this type of response. The neonatal cellular immune response does not seem to be affected by a high level of maternal humoral immunity, so maternal antibodies only have a minimal effect on T cell response, as seen with the Th1-type immune response generated in newborn babies after vaccination against the tuberculosis bacillus. This is believed to be because CD4 T cell responses are not inhibited, unlike the effect on B cells that has already been discussed. Finally, the cellular response in the newborn could in theory be inhibited by maternal cellular immunity, but in practice it is quite rare. In this respect, the cellular immune response to *M. hyo* in piglets originating from sows vaccinated against this pathogen was very similar to those that were not vaccinated, when measured using two different methods (Figs. 19 and 20).

**Figure 19.** Cellular immunity to *M. hyo* measured by the proliferation of mononuclear cells in the blood at (a) 7 and (b) 14 days after vaccination (Vp) or no vaccination (Np) in piglets born to vaccinated (Vs) or non-vaccinated (Ns) sows. Groups with different letters indicate statistically significant differences ($p < 0.05$) (Bandrick et al., 2014).

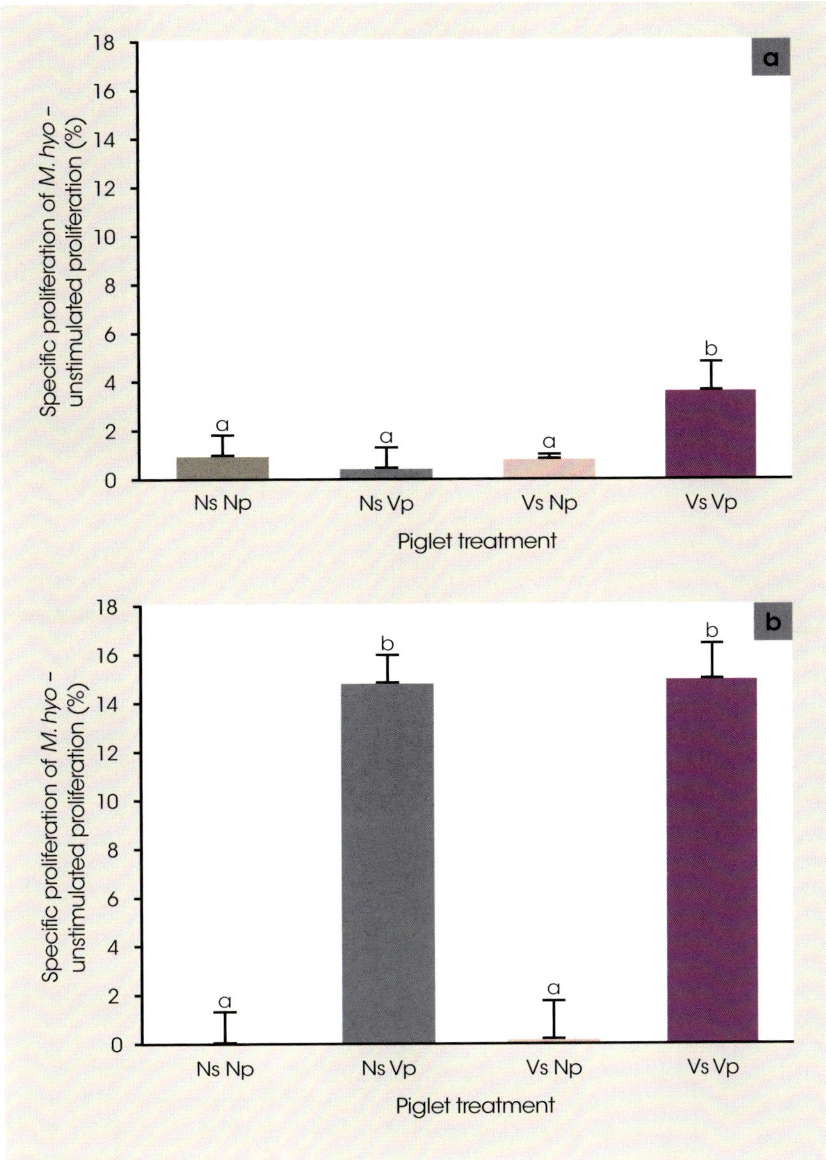

**Figure 20.** Cellular immunity to *M. hyo* measured by intradermal skin testing at (a) 7 and (b) 14 days after vaccination (Vp) or no vaccination (Np) in piglets born to vaccinated (Vs) or non–vaccinated (Ns) sows. Groups with different letters indicate statistically significant differences ($p < 0.05$) (Bandrick et al., 2014).

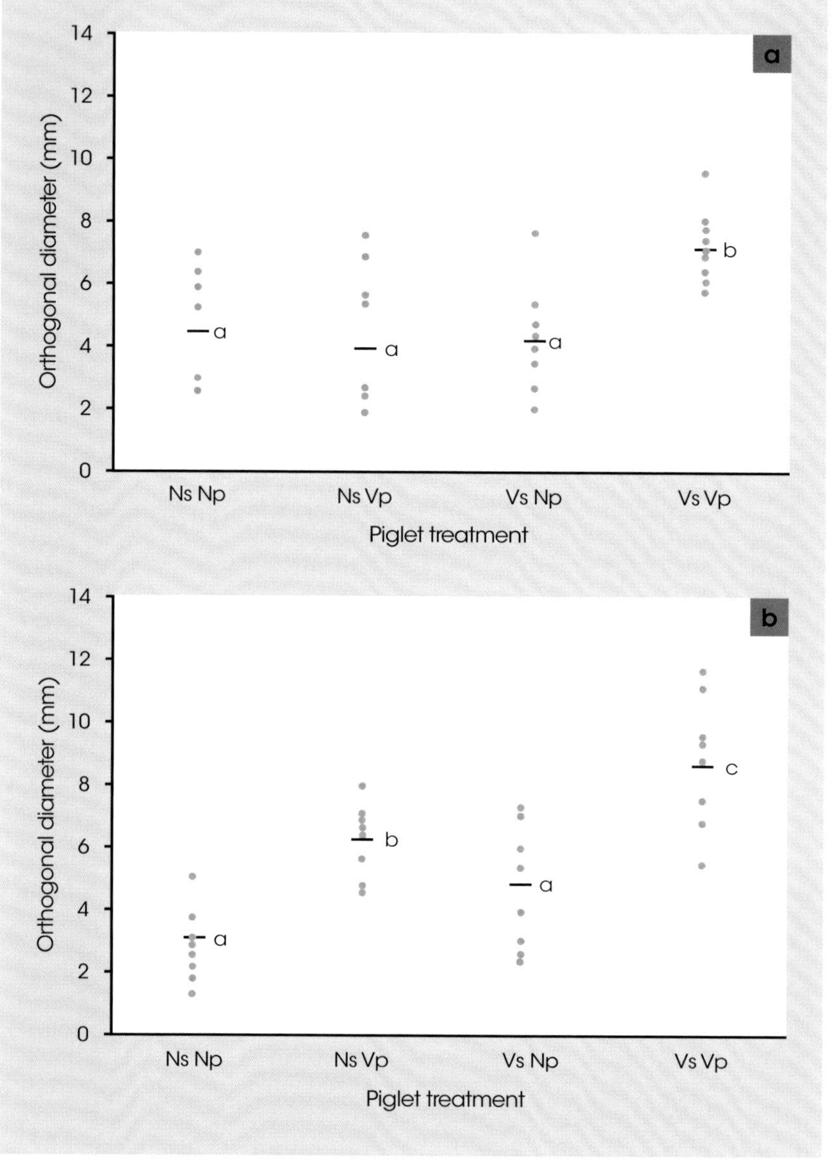

## STRATEGIES TO OVERCOME MATERNAL IMMUNITY AND DEVELOP EFFECTIVE ACTIVE IMMUNITY IN THE NEWBORN

Despite the immaturity of the immune system in very young animals, there can nevertheless be an adequate immune response to vaccination because the immune system in these animals is sufficiently developed to generate, over a period of time, antibodies and memory T and B cells in response to appropriate combinations of vaccine antigens and adjuvants. In fact, many vaccines are designed to be administered to very young animals. A successful vaccine formulation should be able to evade or overcome the functional peculiarities of the neonatal period. Research in this field is centred on modulation of the neonatal innate immune responses to overcome Th1 humoral adaptive immunity by incorporating safe but potent adjuvants into vaccines. In fact, adjuvants are a critical part of pharmaceutical companies' know-how and are protected under patent.

To test the efficacy of a vaccine in the presence of maternal antibodies, (a) maternal antibodies have to be high at the moment of vaccination, (b) the immunological response should be measured by the level of neutralising antibodies and (c) protection should be measured by clinical efficacy, as indicated by the absence of clinical signs or a significant reduction in viral/bacterial loads. This is a requirement for pharmaceutical companies wishing to develop vaccines for very young animals.

Various strategies to minimise the interference of maternal antibodies can be considered in the development of vaccines to be used when these are present.

### Adjuvants

It has been demonstrated that adjuvants in vaccines can minimise this interference. Unfortunately, not much information is publicly available as many adjuvants are protected by patent. However, it is known that inducing type I IFN can strengthen the B cell response in the presence of maternal antibodies via their bond with a surface receptor that stimulates antibody production, even when this pathway has previously been inhibited by maternal antibodies bound to the FcγRIIB receptor (Fig. 21).

### Continuous expression of an antigen or alteration of the antigen

Continuous expression of an antigen relies on obtaining an antibody response through repeated immunisation, even in the presence of maternal antibodies. If a vector system can be designed that continuously expresses the antigen, the B cell responses should be stimulated when the maternal antibody titres have sufficiently reduced. Another strategy involves altering the antigen so that it continues to be immunogenic, and does not inhibit antibody production by the B cells when binding to the FcγRIIB receptor (Fig. 21).

### Alternative routes of administration

Interference can be minimised if the vaccine is administered in an anatomical location with a low IgG titre. For example, if a specific antibody isotype is found in respiratory and ocular fluids, and in the saliva, but at lower concentrations than in the blood, administering a vaccine via the mucosal route can minimise the interference. Various authors have demonstrated that an intranasal Aujeszky's disease vaccine is more effective than a parenteral vaccine in the presence of maternal antibodies. However, there is still some interference, so a booster vaccine is required for vaccination to be effective.

### Vaccines which partially avoid interference

Vector systems have sometimes been used successfully in the presence of maternal antibodies in animal models by using immunisation routes other than the usual subcutaneous or intramuscular routes. Another strategy to overcome interference from maternal antibodies involves the development of DNA vaccines. Various authors have demonstrated that a single vaccination in 8-week-old piglets with a vaccine containing DNA fragments of the Aujeszky's disease virus, namely its glycoproteins gB, gC and gD, triggers a humoral response. This is confirmation that DNA vaccines can overcome interference from maternal antibodies. A memory response has also been clearly demonstrated after secondary DNA vaccination at 11 weeks of age. These data suggest that DNA vaccination in animals with passive immunity successfully generates a strong response. This strategy is very interesting from a scientific perspective, but at present there are no DNA vaccines licensed for use in pigs.

**Figure 21.** Strategies to minimise interference in the development of immunity following the transfer of high levels of maternal antibodies via the colostrum. (a) The antigen is modified so that it cannot interfere with the normal inhibition mechanism. (b) Type I IFN production is stimulated.

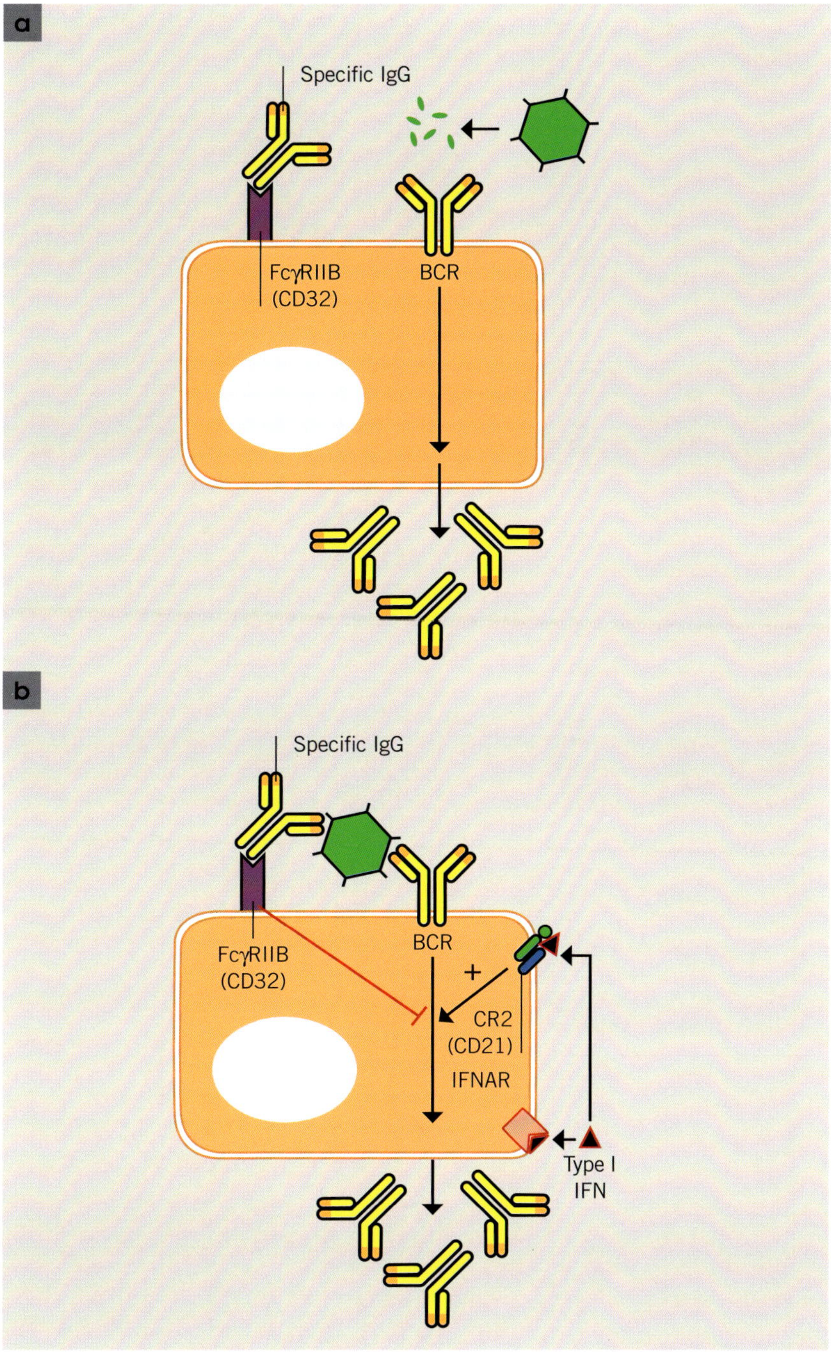

# 04

# PREVENTION PROGRAMMES IN PIGS

# PREVENTION PROGRAMMES IN PIGS

## BASIC CONCEPTS

Pigs are susceptible to a large number of bacterial, viral and parasitic diseases that can limit animal production efficiency. Because these diseases all increase morbidity and/or mortality, increasing production costs and reducing productivity, programmes of preventative medicine are required to minimise the negative effects of these diseases on production, where possible. The preventive medicine strategies that can be used to control diseases were described in Chapter 2, so this chapter focuses on the vaccination of sows to control the main bacterial and viral diseases in pigs. The potential for interference when sows and their piglets are vaccinated against the same pathogen will also be reviewed.

## BACTERIAL DISEASES: SOW VACCINATION PROGRAMMES

The first obstacles encountered by bacteria trying to enter the body are the physical barriers. The first of these is the skin, which prevents these pathogenic organisms from penetrating the body. The mucosae also form a barrier to entry, with their cilia and mucus. There are also many antimicrobial agents in body secretions, such as lysozymes in the saliva. If a pathogenic organism manages to overcome these immune barriers, it will encounter the innate immune system. In the case of bacteria, the most relevant components of the innate immune system are the complement system, using direct bacterial lysis and opsonisation, and NK cells (Fig. 1). Finally, if the bacteria manage to evade innate immune system mechanisms, they will come across the acquired immune system (Fig. 1). Humoral acquired immunity is very important for extracellular bacteria, as it can neutralise the toxins produced by bacteria and facilitate their phagocytosis by macrophages in the extracellular space through opsonisation. Antibodies can also facilitate the phagocytosis and destruction of bacteria in the plasma, which also involves the complement system (Fig. 2). Finally, acquired cellular immunity is critical to develop protective immunity to intracellular bacteria (Fig. 3). *Mycobacterium tuberculosis* and *Brucella suis* are two very important diseases caused by intracellular bacteria in pigs, but they will not be discussed in this chapter, as at present there are no vaccines to control them.

**Figure 1.** Immune response mechanisms to protect the body against bacterial invasion (adapted from Tizard, 2013).

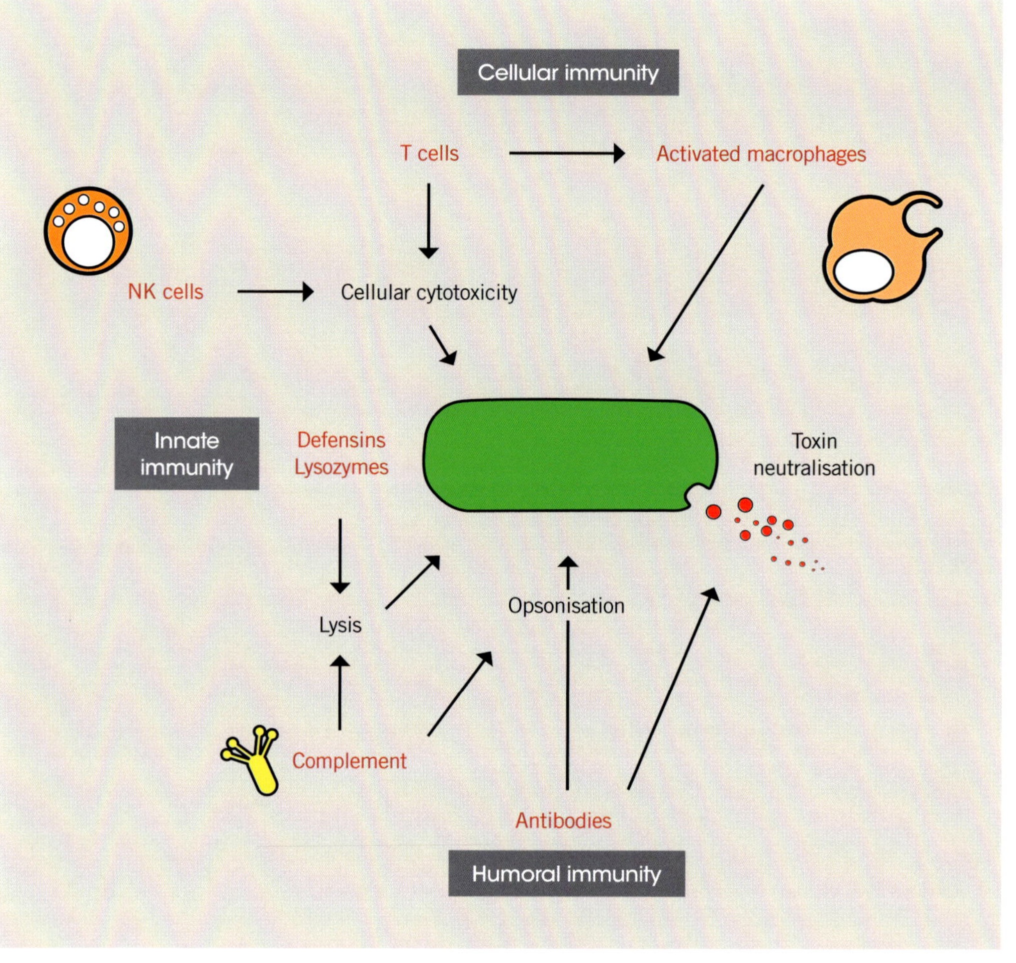

Figure 2. Antibody activity during bacterial infections (adapted from Murphy et al., 2008).

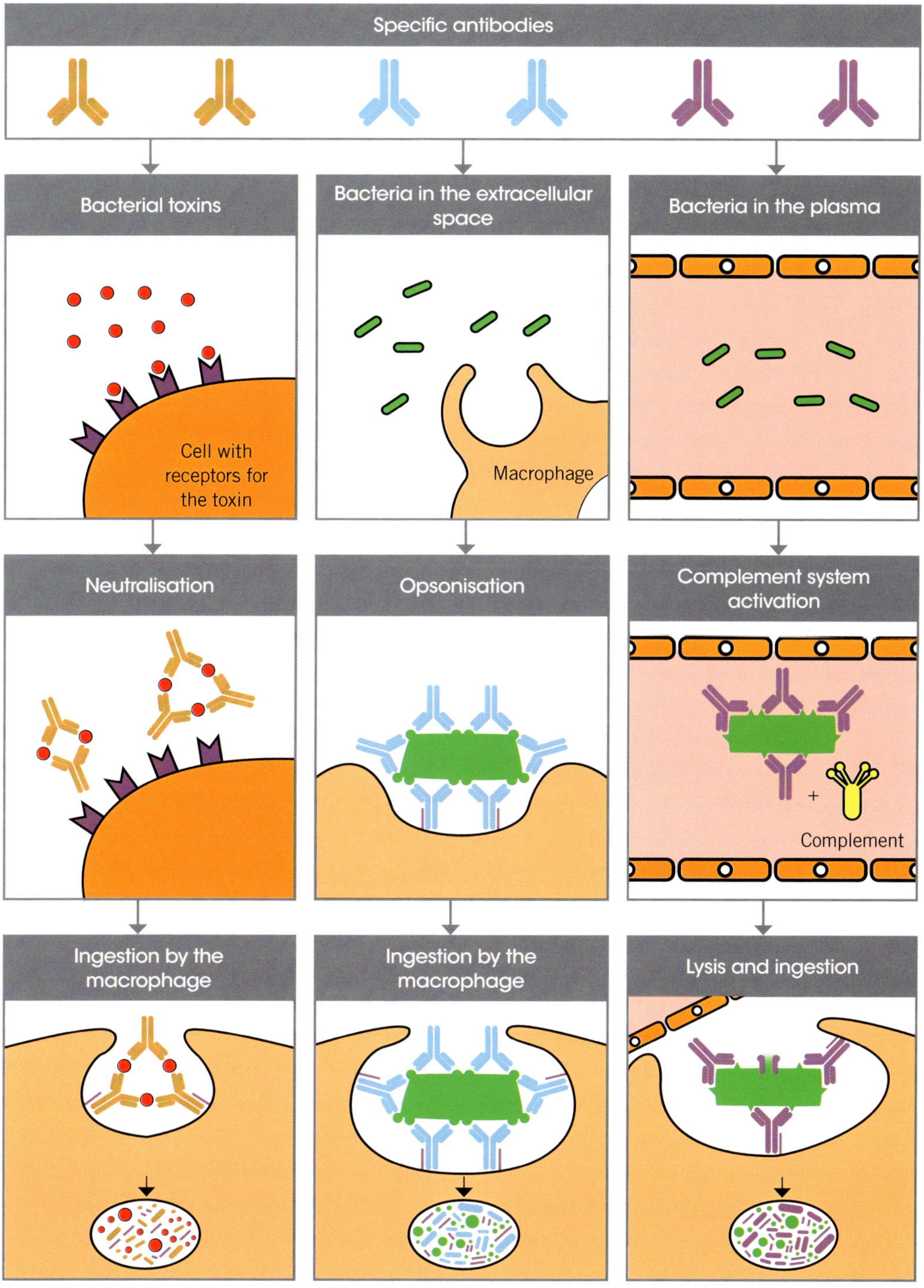

Figure 3. Acquired immune response to intracellular bacterial infections (adapted from Murphy et al., 2008).

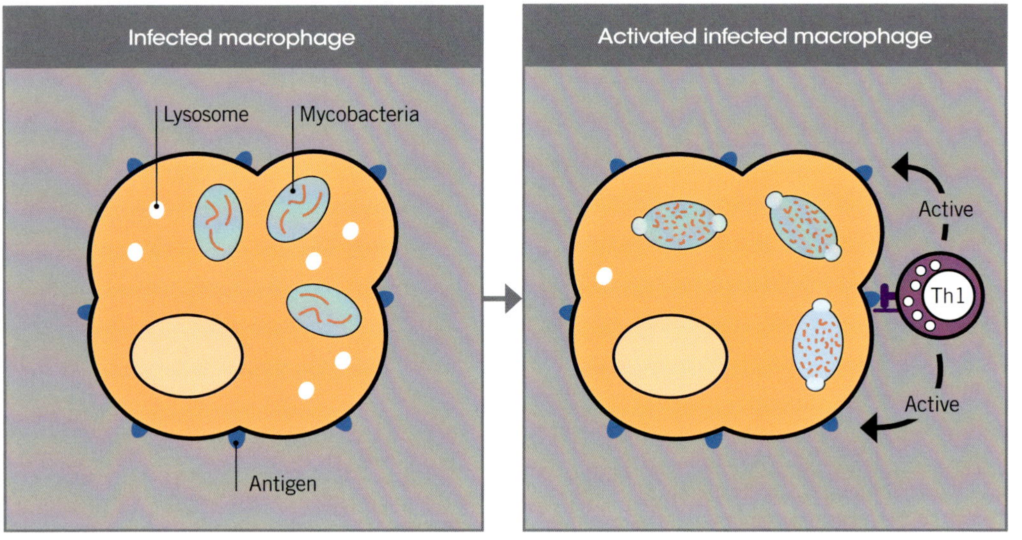


> The vaccines commonly used against bacterial diseases in pigs contain whole inactivated microorganisms (bacterins), purified microbial components or recombinant proteins.

From an antigenic perspective, vaccines against bacterial diseases can consist of attenuated live microorganisms, inactivated bacteria, purified microbial components, recombinant proteins or DNA vaccines. Not all of these vaccines are licensed for commercial use in pigs.

The availability of vaccines containing attenuated bacteria is currently very limited, although two live vaccines are licensed in Europe to control postweaning colibacillosis and porcine ileitis. Historically, vaccine development has been empirical, but advances in microbiology, molecular biology, immunology and bioinformatics have led to a more rational approach to vaccine development. However, many antibacterial vaccines currently used in the field only induce partial protection, so there is still a need to better develop vaccines and vaccination strategies.

## VACCINATION AGAINST EXOTOXIN-PRODUCING BACTERIA

Exotoxins are produced in the bacterial cytoplasm; some toxins are excreted through the cell wall, while others are only released through bacterial lysis, as is the case with *Clostridium* species. The majority of exotoxins are proteins with a high molecular weight, and they usually make powerful antigens. However, there are exceptions, such as the heat-stable enterotoxins produced by enterotoxigenic *Escherichia coli*. These enterotoxins have a low molecular weight and are therefore not very immunogenic.

Antibodies that neutralise toxins are essential to protect the host against diseases caused by exotoxigenic bacteria, as they can prevent the exotoxin from binding to its receptor on the host cell (Fig. 2). So there is reason to hope that disease protection could be gained from vaccines containing an inactivated toxin (toxoid), or an artificial derivative of the exotoxin which is nontoxic but antigenic (recombinant protein). The degree of protection induced by these vaccines is variable and depends on the pathogenesis of the disease.

### Vaccination against clostridiosis

*Clostridium perfringens* is a typical example of an exotoxigenic bacterium. *C. perfringens* isolates are classified into 5 types (A–E), according to their ability to produce the 4 main lethal toxins (α, β, ε and ι). Type A strains of *C. perfringens* are defined by their production of α toxin (although not necessarily only this toxin), while type C strains produce α and β toxins. *C. perfringens* type C has been linked to fatal haemorrhagic necrotic enteritis. This usually occurs in very young piglets, approximately 3 days old, and it can cause very high levels of mortality. The β toxin has a very important role in the pathogenesis of this disease, and neonatal piglets can be protected by vaccinating the sow during gestation with a vaccine containing β toxoid, provided the piglets consume sufficient colostrum. In fact, there are many commercial vaccines on the market that use this toxoid to control porcine neonatal clostridiosis caused by *C. perfringens* type C (Fig. 4). The way in which this toxoid is combined with other antigens in the same vaccine to prevent neonatal colibacillosis will be discussed later.

Isolates of *C. perfringens* type A are linked to enteric diseases in suckling piglets where mild necrotic enteritis is seen. These clinical signs are similar to those caused by *C. perfringens* type C, but mortality is much lower. In both cases, growth slows in these animals, and weight at weaning is therefore lower. Vaccines based on β toxin do not protect against *C. perfringens* type A. Strains of *C. perfringens* type A isolated from piglets with gastrointestinal disease produce β2 toxin, while strains isolated from healthy piglets do not. This β2 toxin is different from the β toxin produced by strains of type C. There is currently a vaccine available in Europe to prevent neonatal clostridiosis caused by *C. perfringens* type A, and the vaccine contains this β2 toxin as the key antigen to confer protection. This vaccine is also administered to gestating sows, and the piglets should acquire enough colostrum to be adequately protected.

**Figure 4.** Preventive medicine strategy to control neonatal clostridiosis in pigs.

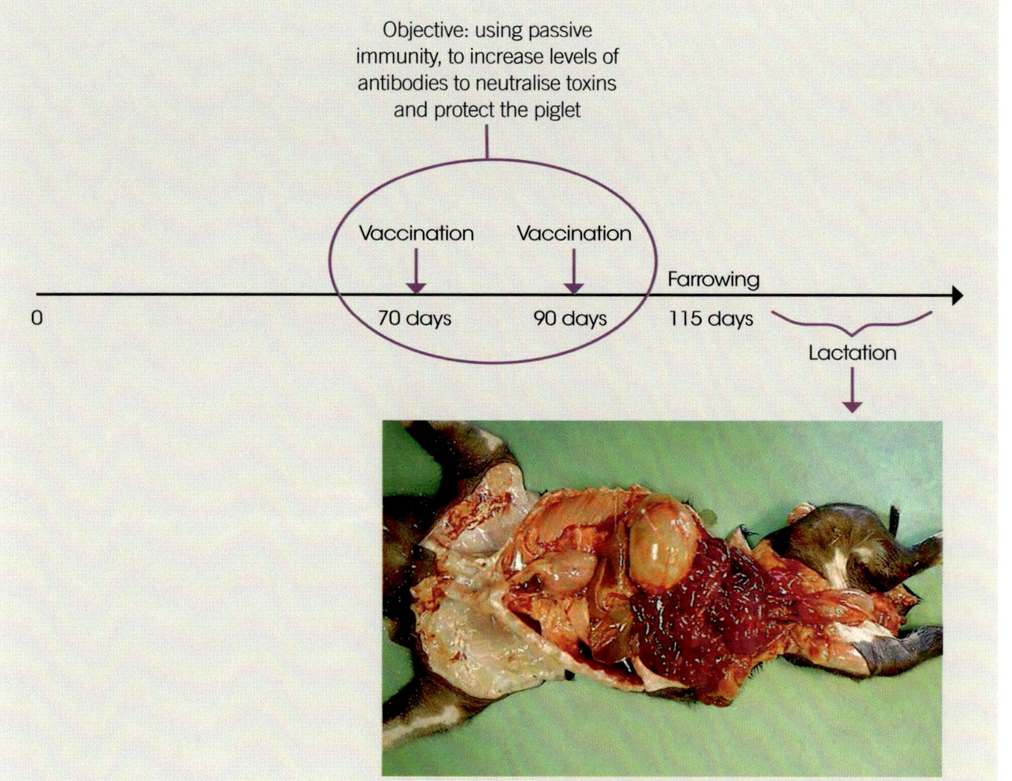


Neonatal clostridiosis: *Clostridium perfringens* type C – β toxin

## Vaccination against colibacillosis

Enterotoxigenic *Escherichia coli* (ETEC) can cause neonatal diarrhoea (in the first few days of life), preweaning diarrhoea (from the first week of age until weaning) and postweaning diarrhoea. ETEC has fimbriae that allow it to attach to specific receptors on the enterocytes. Once attached, ETEC produces enterotoxins that change the flow of water and electrolytes from the small intestine and cause diarrhoea in the piglet (Fig. 5). The four important fimbrial adhesins in neonatal porcine ETEC are F4 (K88), F5 (K99), F6 (987P) and F41. F4-positive is the most prevalent in preweaning diarrhoea in pigs, whereas postweaning diarrhoea is linked to strains of ETEC that produce F4 or F18. ETEC adhering to the intestinal mucosa mainly produces two types of enterotoxin: heat-labile (LT), with a high molecular weight, and heat-stable (STa and STb), which are small, and therefore not very immunogenic, proteins.

Specific antibodies that inhibit bacterial adhesion to the receptors on the intestinal cells and/or neutralise the enterotoxins are

Figure 5. Pathogenic mechanism of enterogenic *E. coli* in suckling piglets.

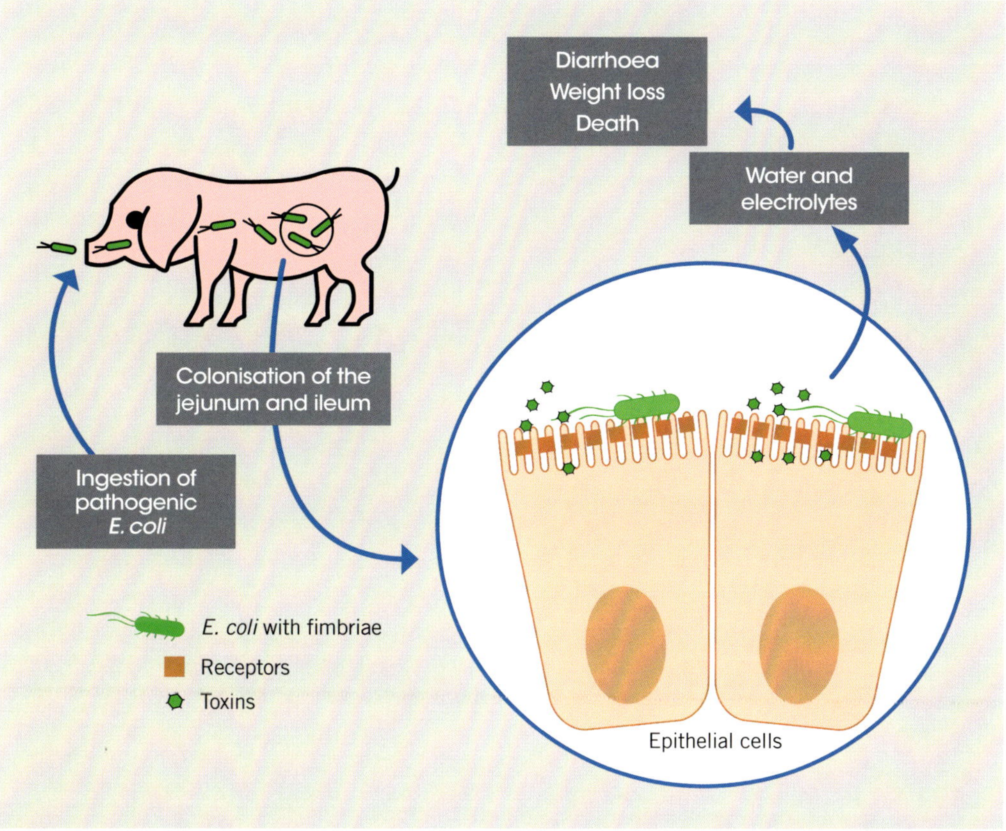


essential to protect against diarrhoea caused by ETEC. Commercially available vaccines are administered by the parenteral route and can be inactivated whole-cell bacterial vaccines or subunit vaccines based on purified fimbriae, which also usually contain LT enterotoxin. These can prevent the bacteria from adhering to the enterocyte and block the toxin once it has been produced by the bacteria (Fig. 5).

Parenteral vaccination of gestating sows with available vaccines mainly stimulates serum antibody production and this is concentrated in the colostrum. Local immunity in the intestines is not stimulated, so IgA levels in milk do not increase. Commercial vaccines are mainly effective against neonatal ETEC diarrhoea, provided that the vaccine contains all the important fimbrial antigens, the piglets consume enough colostrum and infection pressure is not too high. These vaccines are not effective against postweaning diarrhoea, as different fimbriae are involved and the immunity in the intestinal lumen that was acquired through colostrum and milk ingestion has been lost.

## Vaccination against progressive atrophic rhinitis

Progressive atrophic rhinitis is an important disease of the upper respiratory tract in pigs. Characteristic lesions include hypoplasia of the turbinate bones, facial distortion and nasal haemorrhage due to frequent sneezing (Fig. 6). It also causes very significant financial losses to the pig production system, due to retarded growth.

*Bordetella bronchiseptica* and toxigenic strains of *Pasteurella multocida* type D cause atrophic rhinitis in pigs. Infection by toxigenic strains of *P. multocida* causes a more severe and chronic form of the disease, known as progressive atrophic rhinitis, while infection by *B. bronchiseptica* alone is called nonprogressive atrophic rhinitis and has a much smaller effect on growth rate than the progressive type. Infection by *B. bronchiseptica* predisposes pigs to infection with *P. multocida*, and coinfection by both agents causes progressive atrophic rhinitis. Almost all strains of *B. bronchiseptica* produce a dermonecrotic toxin that differs from the *P. multocida* toxin and is responsible for nonprogressive atrophic rhinitis. Various studies have demonstrated that the *P. multocida* toxin is the main virulence factor responsible for the atrophy of the turbinate bones seen in the progressive form of the disease. However, the dermonecrotic *B. bronchiseptica* toxin is also involved in coinfection, so some vaccines also contain the toxoid produced by *B. bronchiseptica*. In any case, antibodies to *P. multocida* and *B. bronchiseptica* toxins have been linked to a lower incidence/prevalence of progressive atrophic rhinitis. Bearing in mind the epidemiology of this disease, active vaccination of sows for passive protection of their progeny is a very controversial way of combating the disease, so the commercial vaccines available contain the *P. multocida* dermonecrotic toxin, an inactivated strain of *B. bronchiseptica* and, in some cases, the *B. bronchiseptica* toxoid. Finally, it is advisable to vaccinate females 6 and 2 weeks before their first farrowing, and thereafter, from the second cycle onwards, at 3 weeks before farrowing (Fig. 6). Vaccination of sows tends to be sufficient to prevent atrophic rhinitis from developing in the piglets during the fattening period. It is obvious that this immunity acquired through the colostrum will not last for the whole of the pig's life, but these antibodies alter the epidemiology of the disease and potentially reduce *B. bronchiseptica* and *P. multocida* colonisation in the piglet population. This is a plausible explanation for how vaccination of the sow tends to be sufficient to control this disease without the need to vaccinate the piglets.

**Figure 6.** Epidemiology and control of porcine atrophic rhinitis.

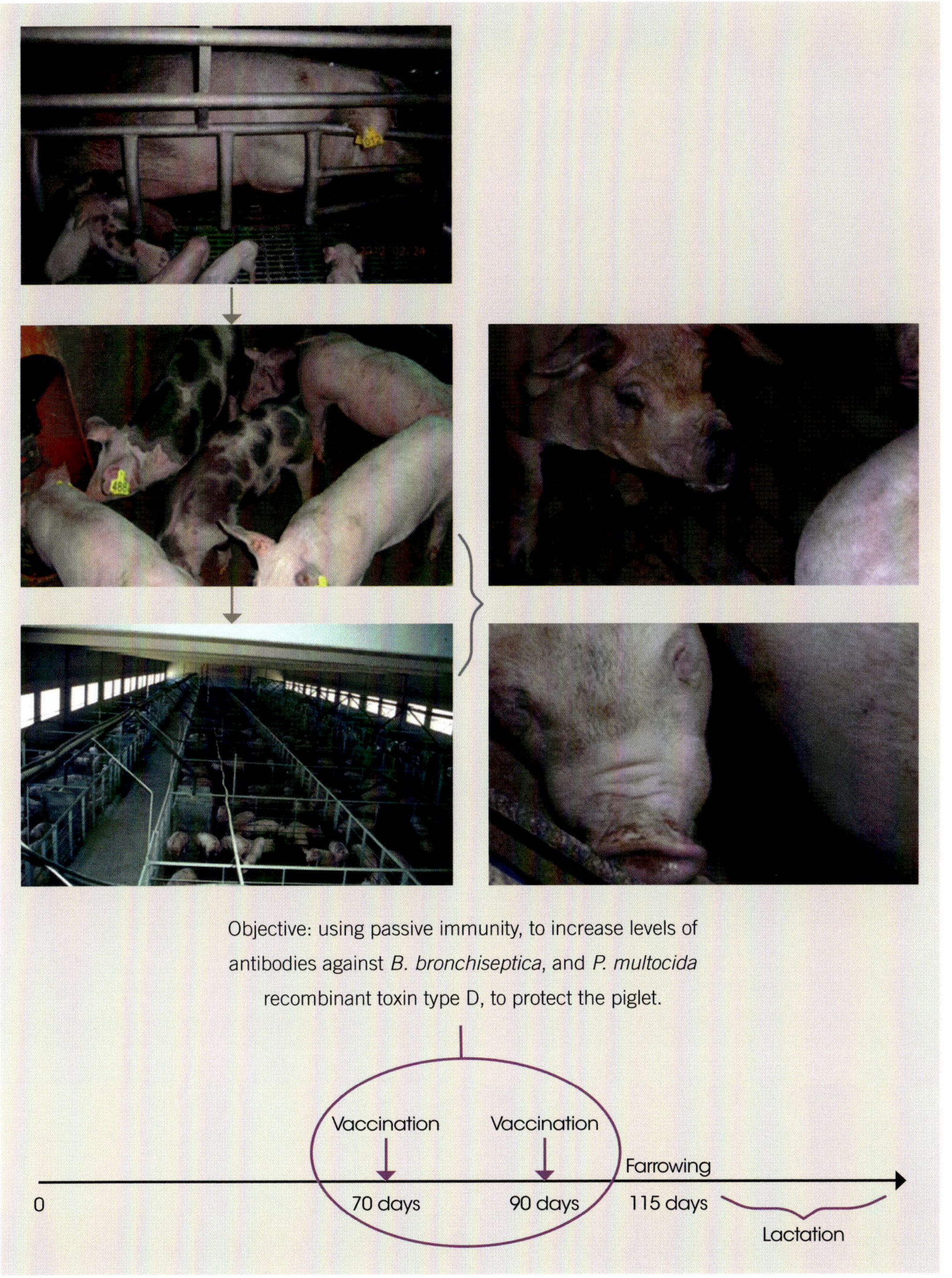

## Vaccination against actinobacillosis

*Actinobacillus pleuropneumoniae* (APP) is the causative agent of porcine actinobacillosis (contagious pleuropneumonia). The disease is found worldwide and causes severe losses to the pig industry. The bacteria can be found in the tonsils of animals that are not suffering from the disease, as a carrier state. There are also a large number of serotypes of very variable virulence. The pathogenesis of actinobacillosis is complex and a large number of virulence factors have been described. *A. pleuropneumoniae* enters the lungs through inhalation and adheres preferentially to the cells of the lower respiratory tract, such as the ciliated cells in the terminal bronchioles, and the alveolar epithelial cells. The disease is characterised by a necrotising haemorrhagic pneumonia and fibrinous pleuritis. Some of the main virulence factors are the exotoxins ApxI, ApxII and ApxIII, that can lyse alveolar epithelial cells, endothelial cells, red blood cells, neutrophils and macrophages. All virulent strains of *A. pleuropneumoniae* express one or two of these toxins. Production of a fourth toxin (ApxIV) by all strains of *A. pleuropneumoniae* has been demonstrated, but its role in pathogenesis is not clear. This fourth toxin is useful in monitoring whether an animal has been infected by this bacterium.

Whole-cell bacterins can reduce mortality after infection by a matching, homologous, serotype, but they do not usually provide protection against heterologous serotypes. This limited protection could be explained by the absence of exotoxins or virulence factors in the vaccine or the presence of antigens that could reduce the efficacy of other antigens in the vaccine. Subunit vaccines containing ApxI, ApxII and ApxIII exotoxins are currently available. These vaccines provide better cross-protection than bacterins, and can reduce clinical signs and improve animal performance. Various studies have shown that *A. pleuropneumoniae* exotoxins are essential components of vaccines to provide protection against infection, but they are certainly not the only factors involved in protective immunity. Vaccines based mainly on *A. pleuropneumoniae* toxins induce partial clinical protection, whenever the challenge dose is not too high, so it is thought that vaccines should include all the virulence factors responsible for the adhesion phenomenon. The problem is that these factors have not been very well characterised, and various antigens are very probably involved.

From an epidemiological perspective, sows are carriers and can transmit the bacteria to their progeny during lactation (Fig. 7). In this phase, the sow transmits the bacteria and the piglet has antibodies acquired from the colostrum that protect against the bacteria. Antibodies protect the piglet from the clinical disease, but there are always a number of piglets whose tonsils have been colonised by weaning (Fig. 7). During the transition phase, the number of animals carrying *A. pleuropneumoniae* in their tonsils gradually increases, and a rapid increase can be seen as levels of maternal antibodies diminish at around 9 weeks of age (Fig. 7). In summary, although sows are asymptomatic carriers, controlling transmission from the sow to the piglet is critical to controlling the disease in growing animals. Subunit vaccines do not tend to be administered to sows for practical

**Figure 7.** Epidemiology of APP infection.

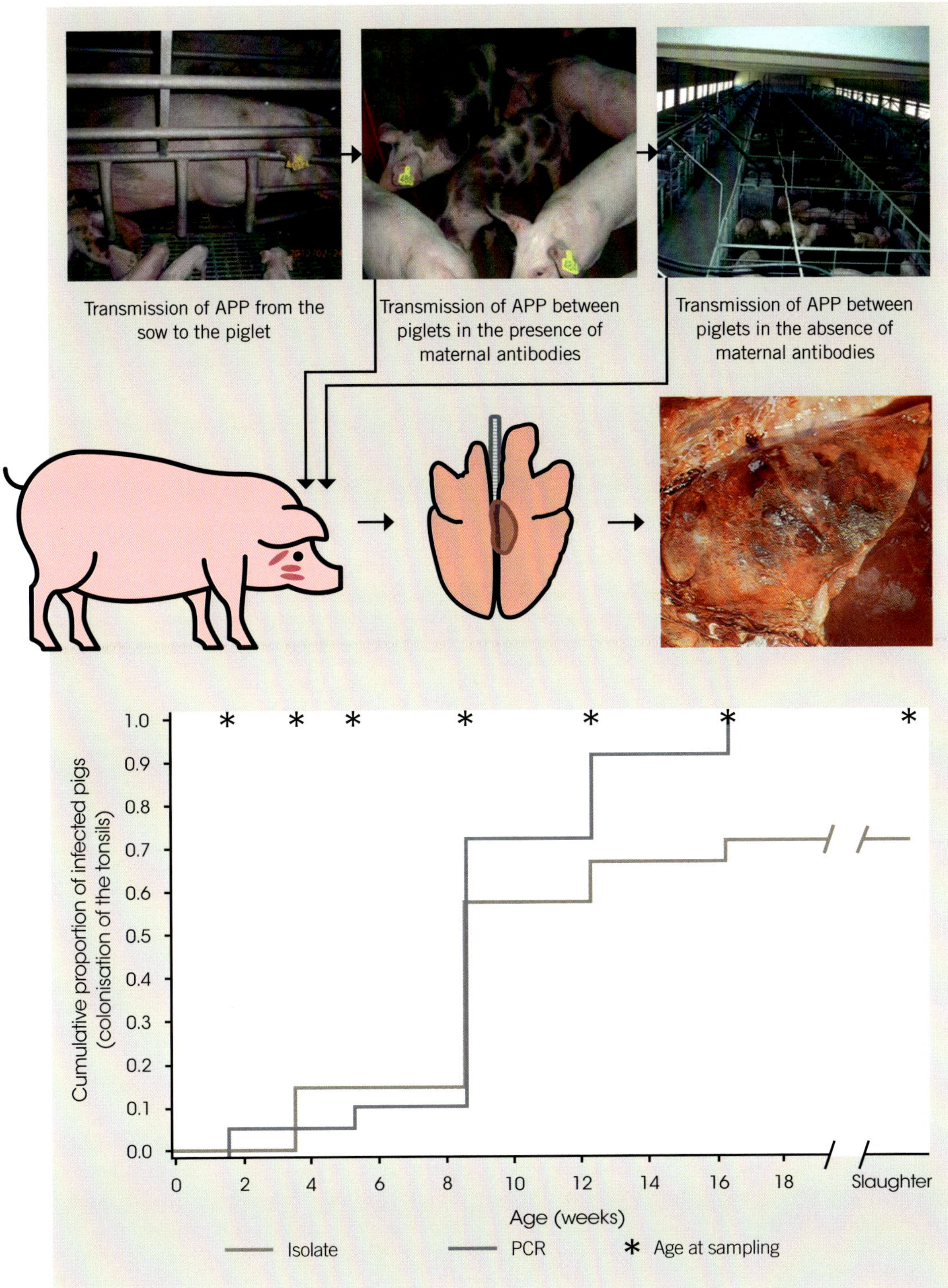

reasons, as these animals are asymptomatic. However, administering bacterins to females during gestation may be a useful tool in controlling the prevalence of piglets carrying *A. pleuropneumoniae* in their tonsils. For this method to be effective, the particular serotype found on that farm must be used.

One of the most common strategies to control *A. pleuropneumoniae* is to vaccinate the piglets with subunit vaccines (*A. pleuropneumoniae* exotoxins) that are active against all serotypes of the bacterium. It is very important to consider any possible interference from maternal immunity in this case, so the first vaccination based on *A. pleuropneumoniae* toxins tends to be recommended from 6 weeks of age. However, there is ample evidence to suggest more lasting interference from maternal immunity, depending on the immune status of the sow, so it is advisable to postpone vaccination of the piglets until 10 and 14 weeks old (Fig. 8). Subunit vaccines also tend to provide immunity for approximately 13 weeks, so animals are protected until the end of their lives if the fattening period has the usual duration.

**Figure 8.** Use of subunit vaccines to control *A. pleuropneumoniae.*

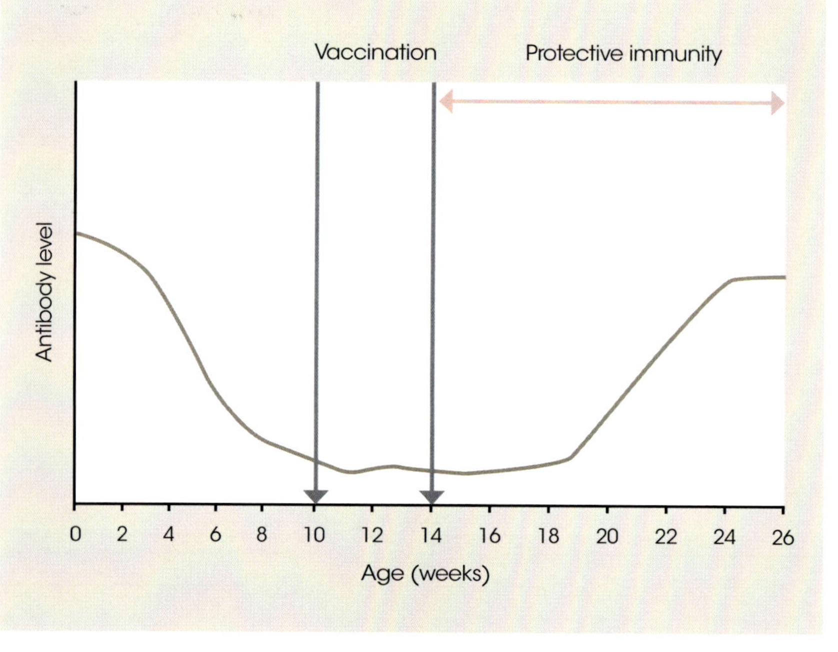

## VACCINATION AGAINST EXTRACELLULAR BACTERIA

Protection against extracellular bacteria is usually mediated by antibodies to their surface antigens and certain secreted antigens. Cellular immunity can also play a role, but it is not considered essential.

### Vaccination against erysipelas

Porcine erysipelas is caused by the gram-positive bacterium *Erysipelothrix rhusiopathiae*. This is a pathogen with 16 serotypes, although clinical disease in pigs tends to be associated with strains of serotypes 1 and 2. It is estimated that 30–50 % of apparently healthy pigs carry *E. rhusiopathiae* in their tonsils and other lymphoid tissues, so there are many carrier animals and predisposing factors are required for the disease to develop. These include environmental factors and stress (e.g. transport or sudden changes to the diet). The disease can be acute, subacute or chronic. Clinical signs of acute and subacute disease are characterised by a generalised infection, and animals tend to develop cutaneous lesions. The pathogenesis of porcine erysipelas is complex and is not fully understood, but it is known that *E. rhusiopathiae* does not produce toxins. However, it is believed that neuraminidase, an enzyme that can cause vascular damage, thrombus formation and haemolysis, is involved in the pathogenicity of the bacterium. The exopolysaccharide capsule (heat-labile) has also been linked to virulence, and it can protect the bacterial cell from host defences, such as phagocytosis. The adhesive surface proteins that bind to proteins in the extracellular matrix are also associated with virulence. The host immune response seems to intervene in the chronic form of the disease. From a clinical perspective, it is very common to see arthritis or endocarditis in animals with the chronic form.

The vaccines used in Western Europe tend to consist of whole inactivated bacteria combined with a soluble immunogen. This latter is produced by selected strains of *E. rhusiopathiae* serotype 2 when it is cultured in a liquid medium. The most active component of this immunogenic product has been identified as a protein fraction with a molecular weight of 64–66 kDa. These vaccines usually provide protection against the acute and subacute forms of erysipelas caused by the common *E. rhusiopathiae* serotypes 1 and 2. However, a slight degree of immune specificity to particular serotypes has been described, so some rare *E. rhusiopathiae* serotypes seem to be refractory to the immunity induced by common vaccines for the disease. This does not seem to be important in clinical practice, as none of these serotypes have been linked to cases of acute porcine erysipelas in the field. The most serious failing of erysipelas vaccines is probably their inability to prevent the chronic form of the disease, so more research is required into the pathogenesis of chronicity.

*E. rhusiopathiae* is an extracellular bacterium, although it can also survive inside cells. Therefore, even though humoral immunity is critical to protect animals, cellular immunity is also involved in protecting against the disease. Maternal immunity also helps protect against erysipelas in very young animals, but maternal antibodies can interfere with the immune response induced by vaccination.

Vaccination against *E. rhusiopathiae* is known to generate protective immunity only when pigs are vaccinated after maternal antibody levels have fallen significantly.

The next section discusses the results of a study that analysed possible interference with the development of humoral and cellular immunity in piglets vaccinated with a live vaccine against *E. rhusiopathiae*. These piglets were either born to sows vaccinated during gestation, or to non-vaccinated sows. In the absence of maternal antibodies, there was no significant difference in mean antibody titres (measured by ELISA) between piglets vaccinated at 6, 8 or 10 weeks of age (Fig. 9b), although only the piglets vaccinated at 10 weeks of age remained above the cut-off point for antibodies to *E. rhusiopathiae* at the end of the study (18 weeks of age). Piglets vaccinated at 6 weeks old became seronegative before those vaccinated at 8 or 10 weeks old. Figure 9a shows the humoral immune response in piglets born to vaccinated mothers. Maternal antibodies remained above the positive cut-off point until 8 weeks of age, and there was no seroconversion in the piglets vaccinated at 6 weeks old; only those vaccinated at 8 or 10 weeks old seroconverted after vaccination (Fig. 9a). These data confirm a high level of interference in the development of humoral immunity in piglets in the presence of very high levels of maternal antibodies to *E. rhusiopathiae*. Indeed, there was a negative correlation between the levels of maternal antibodies at the moment of vaccination and the development of the humoral response after vaccination. This study also quantified cellular immunity by lymphoproliferation assays. In pigs born to non-vaccinated sows, there was proliferation of specific lymphocytes against *E. rhusiopathiae* in all piglets tested 2 weeks after vaccination (Fig. 10). However, at 18 weeks old, there was no longer proliferation in piglets vaccinated at 6 weeks old (NV6), but there were specific antigen responses in 50 % of the animals vaccinated at 8 weeks of age (NV8) and in all pigs vaccinated at 10 weeks of age (NV10). In those born to vaccinated mothers, the specific lymphocytes only proliferated 2 weeks after vaccination in 25 % of piglets which were themselves vaccinated at 6 weeks old (VV6) (Fig. 10). Specific proliferation was seen in all piglets that were vaccinated later than that. Finally, when the piglets reached 18 weeks old, there was proliferation of specific lymphocytes against *E. rhusiopathiae* in 0 %, 23 % and 100 % of the pigs vaccinated at 6 (VV6), 8 (VV8) and 10 (VV10) weeks of age respectively. These results indicate that vaccinating piglets against this bacterium in the presence of high levels of maternal antibodies negatively affects the development of antibodies and the cellular immune response to the disease. Detailed information on this interference should therefore be included in the package inserts for the vaccines available.

**Figure 9.** Humoral immune response to *Erysipelothrix rhusiopathiae* (mean ELISA score ± standard error of the mean) in piglets (a) with and (b) without maternal antibodies before and after vaccination with a single live vaccine against this bacterium. The bold line indicates the positive cut–off point for ELISA. For each group, the first letter refers to maternal status (both gilts and multiparous sows) and the second to piglet status: N = non-vaccinated; V = vaccinated; the numbers following indicate the age of the piglet (in weeks) at the moment of vaccination (Pomorska-Mol et al., 2012).

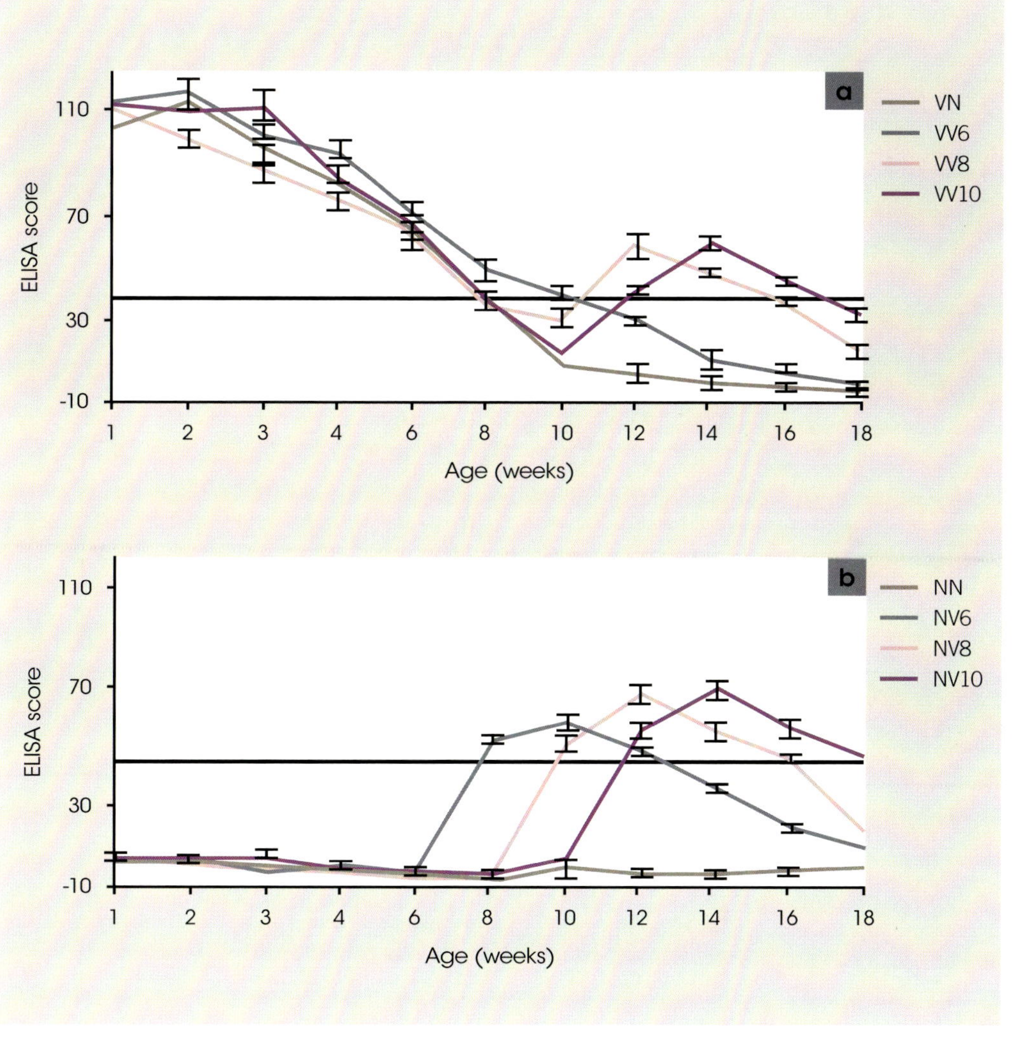

**Figure 10.** Cellular immune response expressed as the mean stimulation index (± standard error of the mean) (a) at 2 weeks after vaccination of weaned piglets and (b) at 18 weeks old. The bold line indicates the positive threshold for specific stimulation of the antigen. For each group, the first letter refers to maternal status and the second to piglet status: N = non-vaccinated; V = vaccinated; the first letter indicates the vaccine status of the mother (both gilts and multiparous sows), the second letter indicates the vaccine status of the piglet, and the numbers following indicate the age of the piglet (in weeks) at the moment of vaccination. The different letters (a–c) indicate statistically significant differences between pigs in the different trial groups ($p < 0.05$), determined by the Kruskal–Wallis test with multiple comparisons (Pomorska-Mol et al., 2012).

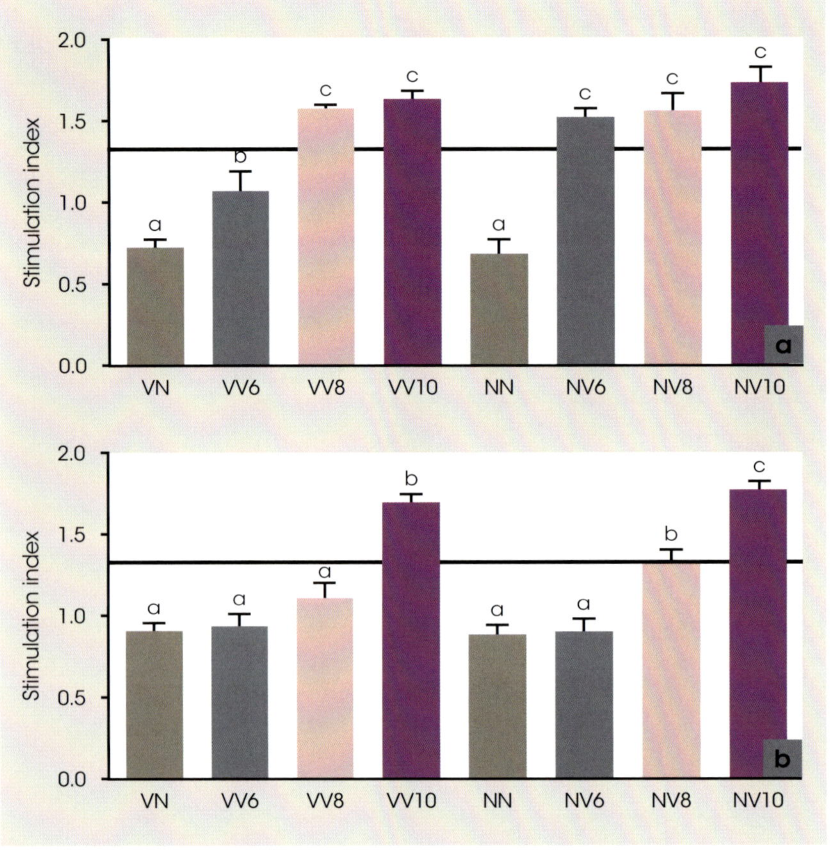

## Vaccination against porcine enzootic pneumonia

*Mycoplasma hyopneumoniae* is one of the pathogens involved in porcine enzootic pneumonia, a chronic respiratory disease that causes significant financial losses to the pig industry. The disease is characterised by chronic coughing and reduced performance in fatteners. The severity of the disease and the financial losses that it causes are very closely linked to concurrent respiratory infections, together with environmental and management conditions. *M. hyopneumoniae* mainly adheres to the ciliated epithelium of the trachea, bronchii and bronchioles, damaging the cells of the cilia and epithelium. The process of adherence, which is necessary before the disease can start, is multifactorial and complex. The interaction between this bacterium and immune function can also be an important factor in the pathogenesis of this disease.

Vaccination with commercial vaccines has become a useful tool to control infections caused by this organism. These vaccines, which are formulated from whole cells plus an adjuvant, have been proven to induce partial protection against the development of microscopic lesions. The exact mechanisms of this protection are not fully understood, but mucosal antibodies and cell-mediated immune responses may be important. Various different vaccination strategies have been adopted according to the type of farm, production system and pattern of infection on the farm. Sows are often vaccinated in the farrowing accommodation, especially when *M. hyopneumoniae* infections occur in the early stages of production. The effect of maternal antibodies on the vaccine response has not been fully established. Piglets with maternal antibodies can show a smaller serological response after vaccination, but the effects on vaccine efficacy are less clear, as levels of serum antibodies after vaccination are not very useful to determine the degree of protection provided by vaccination. In fact, when the cellular immune response in vaccinated piglets born to vaccinated females was measured (Fig. 11), the response was very similar or even better than that of piglets born to mothers that had not been vaccinated against this organism. So all the data available suggests that when vaccinating piglets against this organism, maternal immunity does not interfere with or negatively affect the response that this animal will have to the disease in the future.

## Vaccination against leptospirosis

Porcine leptospirosis, caused by *Leptospira* spp., is a reproductive disease characterised by fertility problems, abortions, or the birth at full term of a variable number of mummified, decomposed, fresh stillborn or weak piglets. Leptospirosis is difficult to diagnose and its prevalence is probably underestimated as clinical signs of infection by *Leptospira* spp. in sows are very variable, from very obvious (uncommon) to vague and nonspecific. This genus of bacteria includes a wide range of species and many of them are not pathogenic in pigs. The species that are pathogenic in pigs (Table 1) are classified into various serogroups and serovars. The Australis, Canicola, Icterohaemorrhagiae and Pomona serogroups belong to the same species (*Leptospira interrogans*), although there is no cross-protection between them.

**Figure 11.** Cellular immunity to *Mycoplasma hyopneumoniae* measured by the proliferation of mononuclear cells in the blood of piglets at (a) 7 and (b) 14 days after vaccination (Vp) or non-vaccinated (Np) born to vaccinated (Vs) or non-vaccinated (Ns) sows. Groups with different letters are statistically significantly different from each other ($p < 0.05$) (Bandrick et al., 2014).

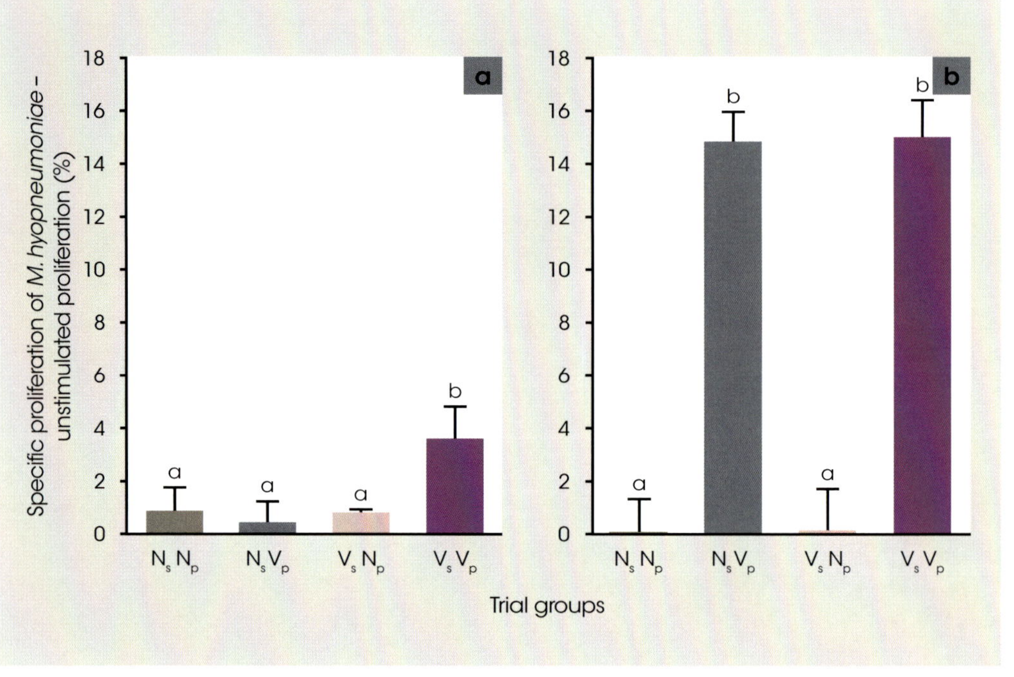


The species *Leptospira borgpetersenii* and *Leptospira kirschneri* are also pathogenic in pigs, and these belong to the Tarassovi and Grippotyphosa serogroups respectively. This point is critical to controlling the disease, as any vaccine should include strains of the 6 serogroups to be effective in all cases. Finally, the inclusion of strains of one of the serovars (Bratislava and Pomona) can be enough to protect against another serovar in the same serogroup (Muenchen and Mozdok respectively). Vaccines are available on the market to protect against *Leptospira* spp. in sows and they all include between 4 and 6 serogroups in their formulation. Young animals do not have to be vaccinated against this disease, so interference from maternal immunity does not have to be considered.

**Table 1.** *Leptospira* species, serogroups and serovars that are pathogenic in pigs.

| Species | Serogroup | Serovar |
|---|---|---|
| *Leptospira borgpetersenii* | Tarassovi | Tarassovi |
| *Leptospira interrogans* | Australis | Bratislava |
| | | Muenchen |
| | Canicola | Canicola |
| | Icterohaemorrhagiae | Icterohaemorrhagiae |
| | Pomona | Pomona |
| *Leptospira kirschneri* | Grippotyphosa | Grippotyphosa |
| | Pomona | Mozdok |

## VIRAL DISEASES: SOW VACCINATION PROGRAMMES

As described for bacteria, the main obstacles that a virus encounters when it tries to enter the body are the physical barriers. If a virus manages to overcome these physical barriers, it will encounter the innate immune system. The most relevant components of the innate immune system against viruses are the complement system (includes lysis of the virus), activated macrophages and NK cells (Fig. 12). If the virus manages to evade innate immune system mechanisms, it will then come across the acquired immune system (Fig. 12). Humoral acquired immunity is important for viruses, as it can inhibit virus adherence to the target cells. Finally, because viruses are intracellular pathogens, any cells infected by them must be destroyed, so acquired cellular immunity is also critical to develop protective immunity to viruses (Fig. 13).

From an antigenic perspective, vaccines against viral diseases can consist of attenuated live microorganisms, inactivated viruses, virus subunits (key proteins for protection), DNA vaccines and vector vaccines. Not all of these vaccine types are licensed for commercial use in pigs.

> The vaccines that are commonly used contain attenuated or inactivated viruses, or virus subunits.

**Figure 12.** Immune system mechanisms to protect the body against invasion by viruses (adapted from Tizard, 2013).

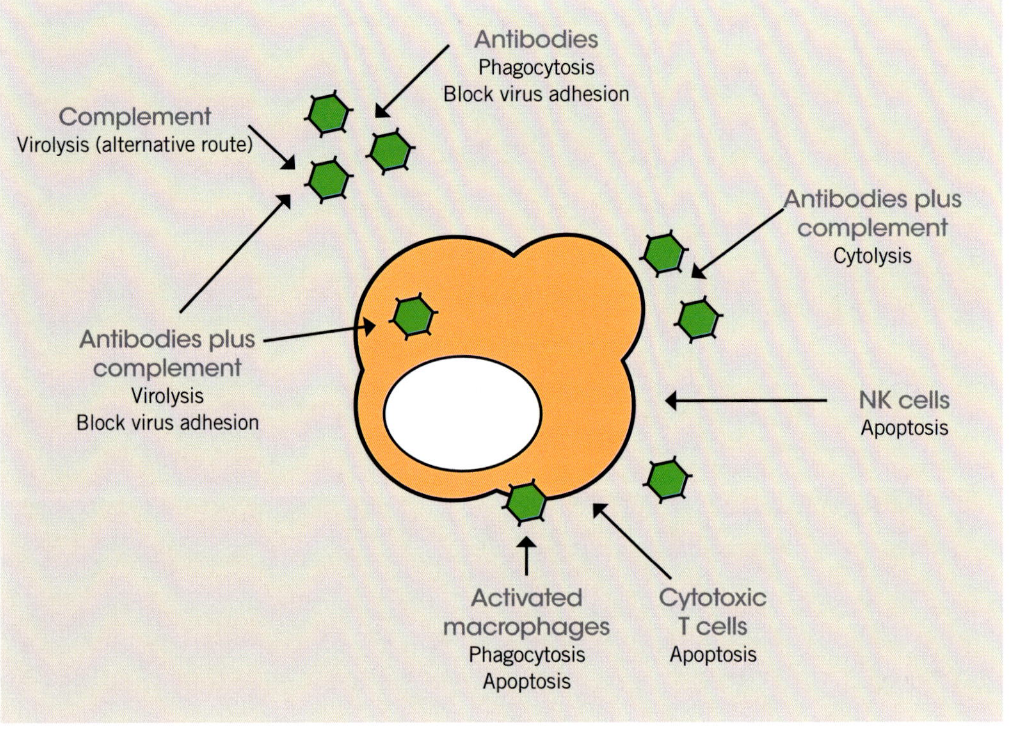


**Figure 13.** Acquired cellular immune response to viral infections (adapted from Murphy et al., 2008).

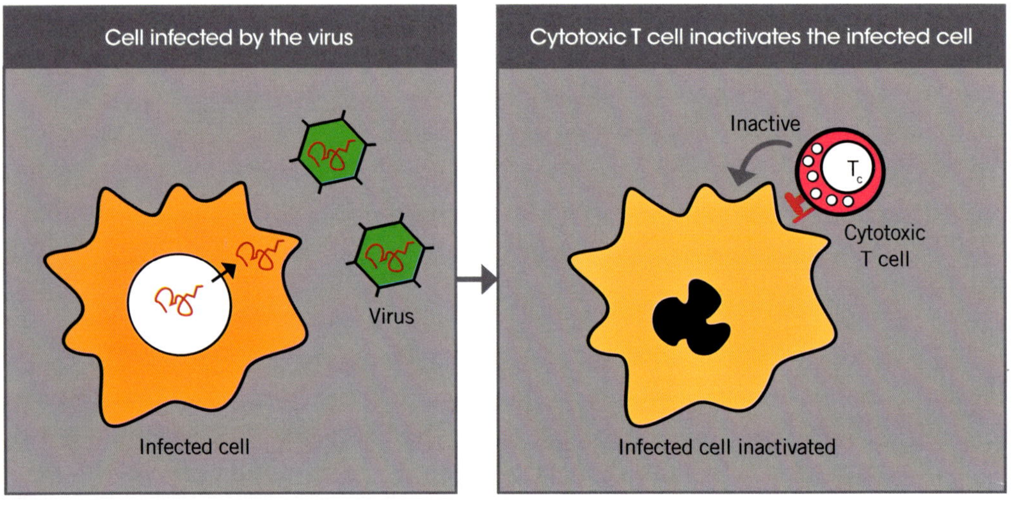

## VACCINATION AGAINST PORCINE REPRODUCTIVE AND RESPIRATORY SYNDROME

Porcine reproductive and respiratory syndrome (PRRS), caused by the PRRS virus (PRRSV), a member of the family Arteriviridae, causes substantial financial losses to the pig industry worldwide. The virus is responsible for reproductive disorders in sows and respiratory problems in pigs during the transition and fattening periods. It can also be a significant factor in coinfections with other pathogens, such as *Mycoplasma hyopneumoniae* and *Pasteurella multocida* for respiratory problems, and *Streptococcus suis* and *Haemophilus parasuis* in systemic diseases.

Modified live PRRSV vaccines (PRRSV MLV) have proven effective at limiting the clinical consequences of infection by this virus, and capable of significantly reducing transmission of the virus under experimental conditions. Therefore, attenuated PRRSV vaccines could be used to control the spread of PRRSV in herds where the disease is widespread, and even to eradicate the virus, both at a farm level and as part of a regional programme to control the disease. However, the ability of attenuated live virus vaccines to control transmission of PRRSV seems to be much lower in practice than under experimental conditions. Despite not understanding precisely either the exact immune response required to protect against the disease, or the type of heterologous cross-protection that may exist between vaccine strains and field strains, attenuated vaccines are widely used to generate immunity to this disease in the breeding sow population. The use of attenuated live virus vaccines in piglets is much more controversial, for three fundamental reasons:

- It takes at least 4 weeks for these animals to develop protective immunity after vaccination.
- There is a great deal of virus recirculation during the transition phase (3–9 weeks of age) in pigs, so protective immunity is only attained if recirculation occurs at the end of the transition phase.
- Potential interference between maternally acquired immunity and live attenuated virus vaccine.

With respect to the last point above, the specific neutralising antibodies to this virus (PRRSV NAs) that are transferred from the mother to her piglets in the colostrum are known to be able to delay PRRSV infection in the piglets. If these levels of passively transferred antibodies are high enough, it has been demonstrated that they are capable of actually preventing PRRSV infection in piglets. The data available suggest that the neutralising antibodies transferred in the colostrum are likely to interfere with the development of active immunity to this virus when piglets are vaccinated with the attenuated live vaccine.

A recent study examined the potential interference between high levels of neutralising antibodies in colostrum produced by vaccinated sows, and the generation of an immune response after vaccination with an attenuated vaccine in their piglets at 3 weeks old. The piglets were vaccinated at this age because this is when vaccines are usually administered (e.g. *Mycoplasma hyopneumoniae* and circovirus vaccines). The distinction between piglets with low (A-) and high (A+) titres of neutralising antibodies was based on serum neutralisation results at one week of age, i.e. on the level of neutralising antibodies to PRRSV, and not by the ELISA results, that detect antibodies to the nucleocapsid antigens. Although this antibody response can be detected by ELISA very quickly after infection, these antibodies to the nucleocapsid antigens do not protect the animal against new infection; they are only useful in indicating past exposure to the virus or passive transfer through the colostrum. After vaccination, the viraemia caused by the vaccine and the humoral and cellular immune responses in the piglets with few maternal antibodies (A-V+) proceeded as described in the literature. Viraemia was thus detected in many of the piglets in this group 2 weeks after vaccination. An early antibody response was also detected by ELISA at the same time. A post-vaccination cellular immune response, characterised by the number of cells producing IFN-$\gamma$, also appeared rapidly. Conversely, neutralising antibodies were detected later, about 4 weeks after vaccination. In contrast, the group that had the highest levels of maternal neutralising antibodies (A+V+) at vaccination failed to show viraemia (from the vaccine), and no immune response was detected during the 4 weeks post-vaccination. It is very reasonable to think that sufficiently high levels of neutralising antibodies at vaccination might act against viraemia by neutralising virus replication, thus inhibiting the immune response to the vaccine. As described previously, in addition to humoral immunity other immune factors, such as cytokines and immune cells, can be transferred in the colostrum. In the study mentioned above, the A+V+ piglets not only differed from A-V+ in humoral status, but also in cellular immune status at vaccination, so the possibility that these cells play a complementary role against the vaccine virus, in addition to the neutralising antibodies, cannot be ruled out. This study was very valid in its specific context, but care must be taken when trying to extrapolate these results to all cases, as this virus is extremely variable, both from a genetic and antigenic perspective, and with respect to the animal's immune response to it. Other studies have actually enabled vaccines for this virus to be licensed for use in Europe for piglets from 2 weeks of age, so it may not be possible to extrapolate the interference seen in this study to all cases, or to all vaccines available on the market. It is therefore very important to discuss this issue with the technical department of the pharmaceutical laboratory that holds the licence for these vaccines. This is all the more relevant because the animals in the study described above were not challenged naturally or experimentally by a field strain of the virus after vaccination. Further research is undoubtedly required to confirm whether the effect of maternal antibodies can endanger vaccine efficacy after challenge with field strains. The effect of antibodies on the ability of a vaccine to protect against disease with respect to not just virological but clinical parameters must be considered. With this particular virus there is no clear correlation between the immune response generated and actual protection, which absolutely must be considered. Finally, from an epidemiological perspective, in order to implement an effective control programme, it is essential to assess the effect of maternal antibody levels on virus transmission and propagation in a vaccinated and subsequently challenged population.

## VACCINATION AGAINST PORCINE CIRCOVIRUS DISEASE

Porcine circovirus type 2 (PCV2) is considered to be the viral agent for PCV2-systemic disease (PCV2–SD), and causes significant financial losses in the pig industry worldwide. PCV-SD was first described in Europe in Spain in 1997 and Denmark at the end of 2001. The disease is now recognised as just one of several diseases associated with PCV2, but it continues to be the most important from a financial perspective. PCV-SD mostly affects 2- to 4-month-old piglets, although it has also been described in animals of other ages. The internationally accepted criteria for PCV-SD diagnosis include compatible clinical signs (mainly wasting and breathing difficulties), moderate to severe lymphocyte depletion with granulomatous inflammation of the lymphoid tissues, with medium to high levels of PCV2 in these lesions. As the virus is ubiquitous and has also been found on farms where no pigs have shown clinical signs of PCV-SD, detection of PCV2 antibodies, and/or viral antigens or DNA in the serum does not constitute a diagnosis of PCV-SD, but only indicates infection with PCV2. This is a clear example of a multifactorial disease where the virus is a necessary prerequisite, but not enough on its own for the disease to develop.

Commercial PCV2 vaccines are a very useful tool to control the diseases associated with this virus. In the field, vaccinating sows increases their serum PCV2 antibody levels and reduces viraemia; it also reduces excretion of the virus in the colostrum and milk. Vaccination also improves production parameters in their piglets by reducing the mortality rate and increasing the daily weight gain. It can reduce the incidence of reproductive problems associated with the virus in breeding sows, although this has not been studied very closely and is poorly understood. Vaccines against this virus are therefore licensed for use in sows, and they have been widely used to control the diseases associated with the virus in these animals.

Vaccinating piglets against PCV2 significantly reduces the effect of the diseases associated with the virus in growing animals, which suffer most from the disease. Vaccinating these animals can therefore reduce the proportion of PCR-positive animals at any particular age, and/or delay infection by PCV2. It also reduces the gross lesions associated with the virus and the frequency of coinfections, and improves average daily gains and mortality in fatteners. These effects are achieved by stimulating a humoral and cellular immune response that can protect piglets against this viral infection following vaccination. With this disease, the response required to generate good protective immunity is known. These days, using a PCV2 vaccine for growing pigs is considered ‘universal’, as it yields significant financial return in both clinical situations where PCV-SD is present, and subclinical situations, where viral infection with PCV2 exists, but there is no clinical disease.

As mentioned previously, sows and/or piglets can be vaccinated against PCV2. However, the issue of whether there is interference to the immune response in piglets born to mothers vaccinated against PCV2 still needs to be clarified. Vaccinating sows with a single PCV2 vaccine 1 week before insemination can induce high antibody titres in their piglets at 4 weeks old, and delay PCV2 infection compared with piglets born to non-vaccinated sows (NV-NV) (Figs. 14 and 15). Vaccinating the sows also significantly increased the average daily gain of their progeny, as this parameter was significantly greater in piglets born to vaccinated mothers (V-NV) compared to piglets born to non-vaccinated mothers (NV-NV) when they were between 12–21 weeks old. Antibody titres after vaccination increased in those that had received low levels of PCV2 antibodies via the colostrum (usually born to non-vaccinated mothers [NV-NV]) (Fig. 14), but levels did not

**Figure 14.** Transfer of humoral immunity in vaccinated and non-vaccinated sows. Inverse log2 of the titres obtained by immunoperoxidase monolayer assay (IPMA) (± standard deviation) for the 75 pigs tested per treatment group per sampling session. Different letters in the same table column indicate statistically significant differences ($p < 0.05$) (Fraile et al., 2012).

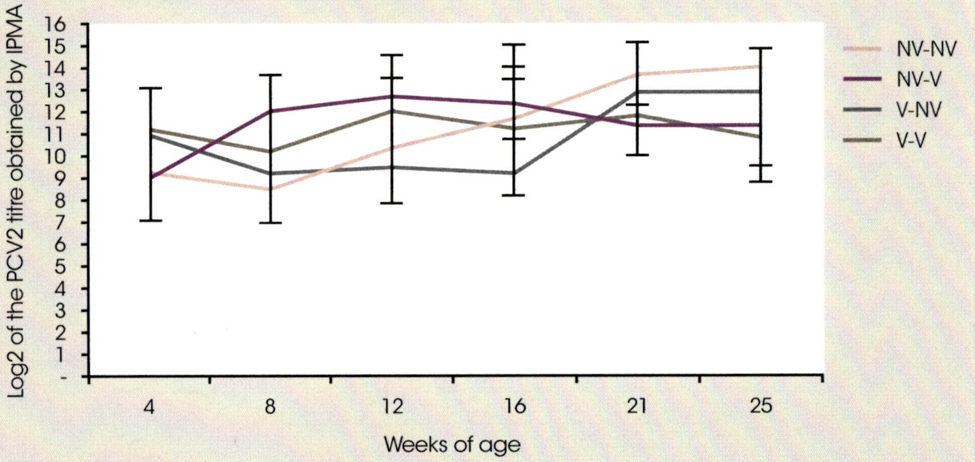


| | Weeks of age | | | | | |
|---|---|---|---|---|---|---|
| Groups | 4 | 8 | 12 | 16 | 21 | 25 |
| NV-NV | b | d | c | a | a | a |
| NV-V | b | a | a | a | c | c |
| V-NV | a | c | c | b | b | b |
| V-V | a | b | b | a | c | c |

increase, and even fell, after vaccination in piglets that received a high level of antibodies via the colostrum (usually born to vaccinated sows [V-V]) (Figs. 14 and 16a). This indicates that there is interference in the development of the humoral immune response. Based on these data, it could be assumed that double vaccination (sows and piglets) against PCV2 would have a negative effect on production in these animals. However, this is not the case as the results are very different when analysed from a virological and production perspective. The proportion of animals with PCV2 in their serum, and their productive performance, using mortality rate and average daily gain, is very similar in piglets born to sows vaccinated against PCV2 and non-vaccinated sows (Fig. 16) throughout their entire lives. These results clearly indicate that vaccine efficacy against PCV2 in piglets has been demonstrated even in the presence of maternal antibodies to PCV2 at vaccination.

**Figure 15.** Percentage of PCV2 positive pigs measured by PCR out of a total of 75 pigs tested per treatment group per sampling session. Different letters at the same point indicates statistically significant differences ($p < 0.05$) (Fraile et al., 2012).

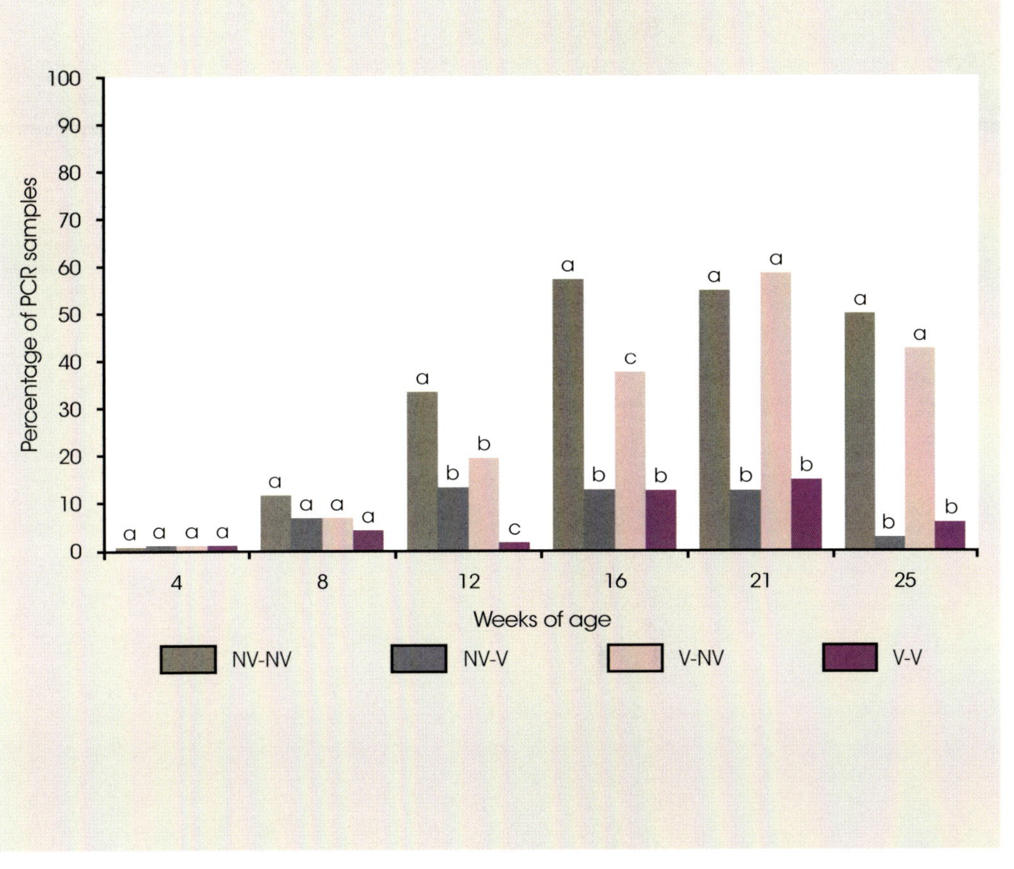

**Figure 16.** (a) Linear regression between the inverse log2 of the PCV2 titres obtained by immunoperoxidase monolayer assay (IPMA) at vaccination (3-4 weeks of age, x-axis) and the increase in these titres from 3-4 weeks to 8 weeks of age (delta value, y-axis) in vaccinated piglets born to vaccinated sows (V-V) and non-vaccinated sows (NV-V). (b) Linear regression between the log2 of the PCV2 titres obtained by IPMA at vaccination (3-4 weeks of age) and the average daily gain (ADG) from 3-4 weeks to 25 weeks of age (Fraile et al., 2012).

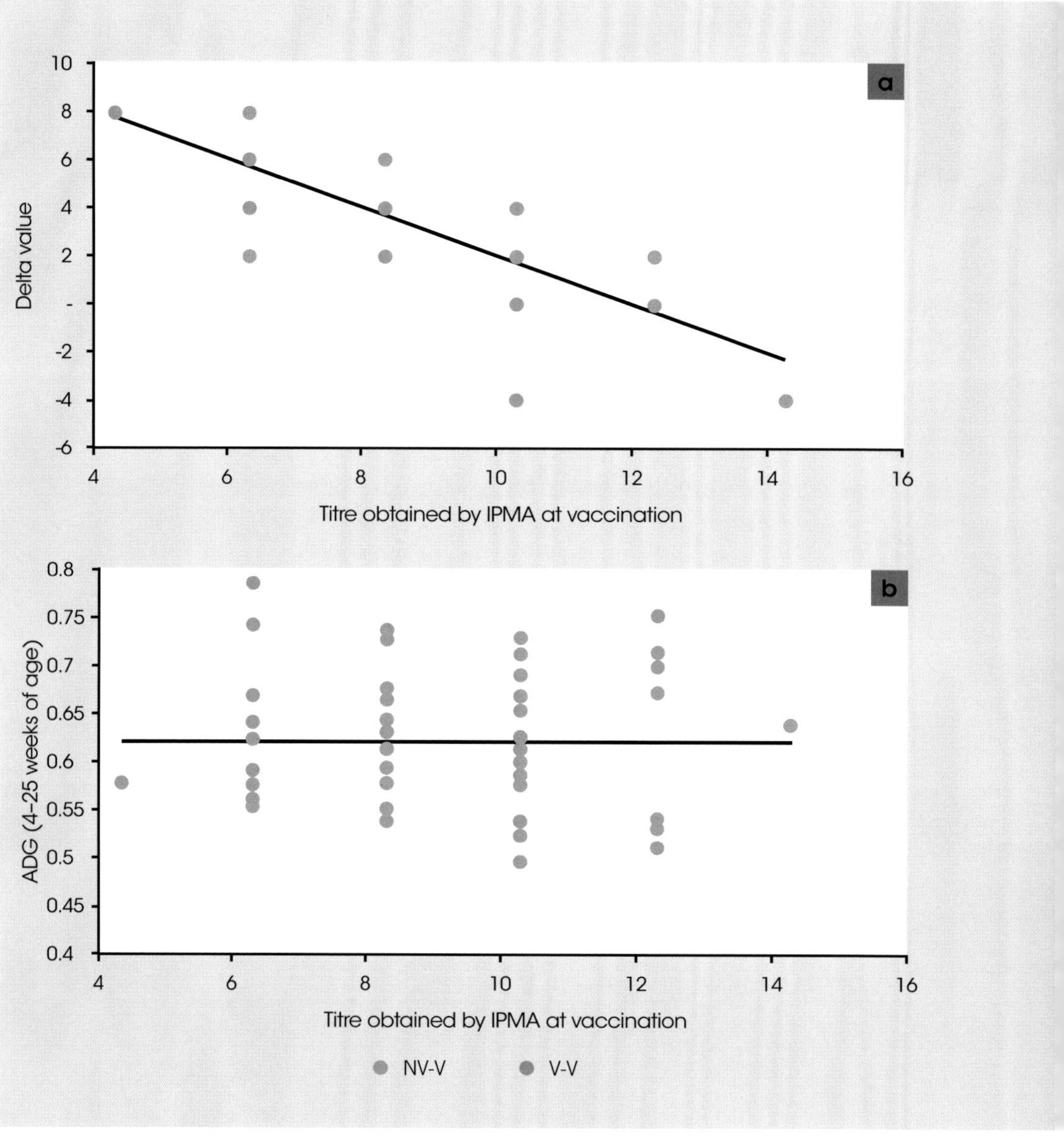

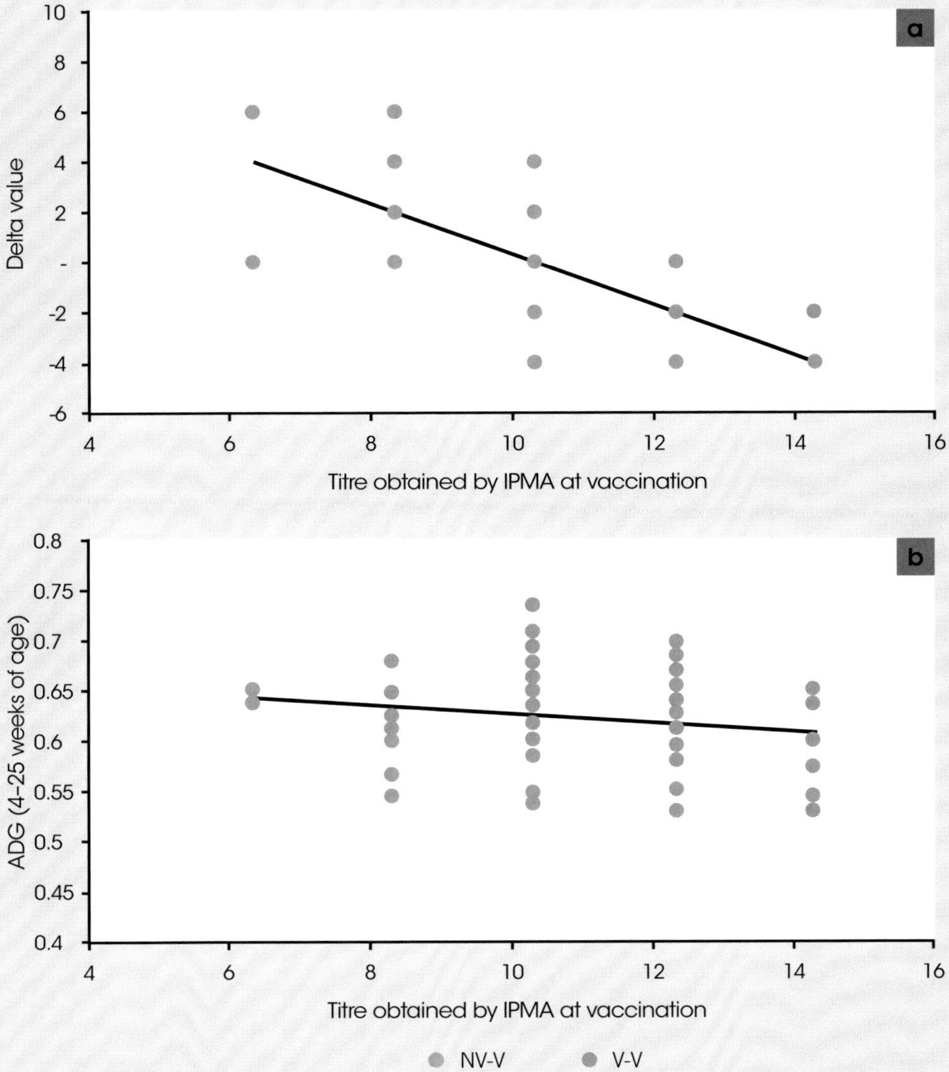
a
Delta value
10
8
6
4
2
-
-2
-4
-6
4
6
8
10
12
14
16
Titre obtained by IPMA at vaccination
b
ADG (4–25 weeks of age)
0.8
0.75
0.7
0.65
0.6
0.55
0.5
0.45
0.4
Titre obtained by IPMA at vaccination
NV-V
V-V

## VACCINATION AGAINST PARVOVIRUS INFECTION

Porcine parvovirus, renamed ungulate protoparvovirus 1 (UPV1), is a member of the genus Protoparvovirus and family Parvoviridae. It is very widespread in the pig population, despite the use of vaccines against the virus being routine for many years. It is characterised by causing exclusively reproductive problems. Clinical expression of the disease depends on the pathogenicity of the virus and the sow's stage of gestation, so foetuses infected before 70 days' gestation tend to die, while those infected later develop antibodies to the virus, eliminate it and survive infection. On a farm level, infection by the virus causes reproductive problems that are mainly evidenced by an increase in mummified piglets at farrowing and small litters (due to early embryonic death).

Prevention of infection by this virus is based on vaccinating all replacement gilts before their first service, so this vaccination has become routine in gilt introduction programmes on all pig farms. A booster is also administered to sows 1 week after farrowing to induce a so-called boosting effect before the next service. It has been known for some time that piglet immunity to this virus acquired through the colostrum interferes with the development of immunity following vaccination. A recent study analysed the dynamics of antibodies to porcine parvovirus on commercial farms. The highest level of parvovirus antibodies was detected in piglets after colostrum consumption, and this decreased until 3 months of age, with the half-life of maternal antibodies being 29.8 days. Previous studies have determined that these antibodies can remain until they are 6 months old. Therefore, in practice it is advisable not to vaccinate gilts against this virus before 6 months of age.

## VACCINATION AGAINST SWINE INFLUENZA

Swine influenza is an acute respiratory disease caused by the influenza type A virus (IAV) which belongs to the family Orthomyxoviridae. In pigs, infection by IAV affects the epithelial cells in the nasal mucosae, tonsils, trachea and lungs. There is an influx of neutrophils and other inflammatory cells, which causes necrosis of the epithelial cells and obstruction of the airways. This virus evolves rapidly, so there are currently many different strains circulating together in pig populations. IAVs are classified into subtypes by function of the antigenic differences between the two major surface glycoproteins, haemagglutinin (HA) and neuraminidase (NA). HA subtypes H1 and H3 are currently circulating in pigs worldwide, in association with different combinations of neuraminidase genes (N1 and N2). This combination gives rise to the most prevalent IAV subtypes in pigs worldwide: H1N1, H1N2 and H3N2. However, their origin, gene combinations and antigenic composition vary greatly across the continents. Such variation has led to them being classified by their HA gene into different phylogenetic groups within the H3 (IV-A, -B, -C, -D, -E and -F) and H1 ($\alpha$, $\beta$, $\gamma$, $\delta$1, $\Delta$2 and H1N1pdm09) groups. The natural evolution of IAV is closely linked to the tendency of viral polymerase to generate errors, and to the segmented nature of its genome. The diversity of IAV is also increased by a combination of mechanisms, including reorganisation of gene segments, point mutations and the introduction to pigs of influenza from other hosts, especially humans. Once the virus begins circulating in pigs, this very dynamic IAV population continues to evolve by reassortment, and the antigenic shift continues to shape the evolution of IAVs in this species. Different genetic groups are often antigenically distinct, and limited serological cross-reactivity can be detected even within a group, as well as between different groups. This limited cross-reactivity has proven an obstacle to the development of an effective vaccine.

Infection by swine influenza is often characterised by rapid onset with high fever, lethargy, loss of appetite, laboured abdominal breathing and coughing. The disease lasts 2 to 6 days and although mortality is low and most animals recover, weight loss can be significant. This pathogen contributes to the porcine respiratory disease complex and is occasionally linked to abortions caused by fever in sows. As with any other pig disease, vaccination is a useful tool to control the virus. The virus haemagglutinin protein is the main target for neutralising antibodies. The antibodies that inhibit haemagglutination of the virus in the red blood cells (measured by haemagglutination inhibition [HI] assay) tend to correlate closely with the protection acquired against the disease. Natural infection with this virus tends to develop cellular immunity, which protects against reinfection.

The only swine influenza vaccines available in Europe are based on whole inactivated viruses (WIV) combined with potent adjuvants. These vaccines stimulate strong antibody responses that can be measured by HI, although the cellular response is weak or non-existent (Fig. 17). Viral variants that are not recognised by the antibodies generated by these vaccines can make previously used vaccines ineffective. Therefore, vaccines are more effective if the strains they contain correspond closely to the strains actually circulating in the population at that particular time. In human medicine, precise epidemiological surveillance is conducted to find out which strains are circulating in the population, and the strains included in WIV vaccines are continuously modified. This strategy would also be advantageous in pigs, but European legislation does not permit this flexibility, so the strains used in commercial vaccines cannot be changed before many trials have been carried out by the pharmaceutical companies. Legislation in the United States is more flexible and allows vaccine manufacturers to update the strains in inactivated vaccines to match the current genetic diversity. The use of vector-based (alphavirus) vaccines has also been authorised since 2012 and their characteristics are summarised in Figure 17. This type of vaccine is still not licensed for use in Europe. Finally, it is also possible to use vaccines based on attenuated live viruses, administered intranasally (the natural route of infection). However, this type of vaccine is still only available for experimental use, as there are serious doubts about the safety for on-farm use (potential recombination with the field flu virus). However, they do enable better cross-protection with the viruses that are circulating in the field (Fig. 17). It is worth noting that inactivated vaccines are the most commonly used to control this disease worldwide.

However, sterilising immunity tends to be unattainable with inactivated vaccines for IAV, at least over a period of time, due to the considerable ability of the virus to evolve and evade the host's immune response. Therefore, the more realistic objective is to prevent clinical disease and reduce virus replication and excretion without causing immune-mediated pathology. Many inactivated vaccines are multivalent (contain 2 or 3 different viruses), so it is necessary to investigate whether the response to all the viruses is similar, and sufficient to confer protective immunity, as some viruses are not very immunogenic and induce very low HI titres, even when combined with adjuvants. From a practical perspective, it is very common to vaccinate breeding females to prevent them contracting the disease during gestation and also prevent an increase in the incidence of reproductive problems (abortions caused by fever) in the population. Vaccination against IAV not only provides the sows with immunity, but also transfers passive maternal immunity to the progeny through the colostrum.

Vaccinating breeding females against IAV is common practice in the pig industry, to stimulate the passive transfer of antibodies in the colostrum, using multivalent WIV vaccines. In homologous infections, where the vaccine and challenge viruses are similar, the maternally derived antibodies (MDA) acquired from the colostrum are correlated to the piglet's protection against the clinical disease. However, they do not prevent the animals from being infected or the virus being excreted (Fig. 18), so IAV infection and transmission can occur in the presence of maternal immunity. However, MDA levels reduce virus excretion significantly, to the point where the basic reproduction rate (defined as the number of piglets that are infected by one infected animal in its infectious phase) is much lower in piglets with a high level of maternal immunity than those that have not acquired this passive immunity, when challenged with a homologous virus. These data suggest that homologous immunity cannot prevent transmission completely, but does, however, help reduce and control the disease. However, levels of protection can vary widely according to the strain of the virus, MDA levels and age at infection. The genetic diversity of IAV also makes it difficult for immunity acquired from the sow to cross-protect against heterologous viruses on the farm. Finally, it has been known for some time that MDA levels interfere with generation of the humoral immune response (IgA, IgM, IgG and HI) and the cellular immune response following primary or secondary exposure to the virus (Fig 19). Thus, MDAs can suppress the serum antibody response and induction of a memory T cell response after vaccination against swine influenza. Various studies have confirmed that the presence of MDAs at vaccination reduces vaccine effectiveness, with longer periods of fever and the appearance of clinical signs after infection with the virus. This is why it is not advisable to vaccinate piglets that have high levels of maternally derived humoral immunity with inactivated flu vaccines. In fact, the package inserts recommend vaccinating piglets after 6–8 weeks of age, depending on the vaccines available on the market.

**Figure 17.** The type of vaccine and the route of administration affect the resulting immune response. WIV vaccines are administered intramuscularly, and attenuated live virus (ALV) vaccines are normally administered intranasally. Vector or RNA vaccines can be administered by either of the two routes. The route of administration, and the way in which the vaccine antigens are presented to the immune system affect the host's subsequent immune response.

| | WIV | Vector | LAIV |
|---|---|---|---|
| Route of administration | Intramuscular | Intramuscular/ Intranasal | Intranasal |
| HI response | +++ | ++ | + |
| Antibody-secreting cells | ++ | + | + |
| Memory B cells | + | + | + |
| Nasal IgA | -/+ | -/+ | +++ |
| Antibodies to NA | +++ | -/+ | ++ |
| CD4 T cells | ++ | ++ | +++ |
| CD8 T cells | - | + | + |
| Cross-protective immunity | -/+ | + | ++ |

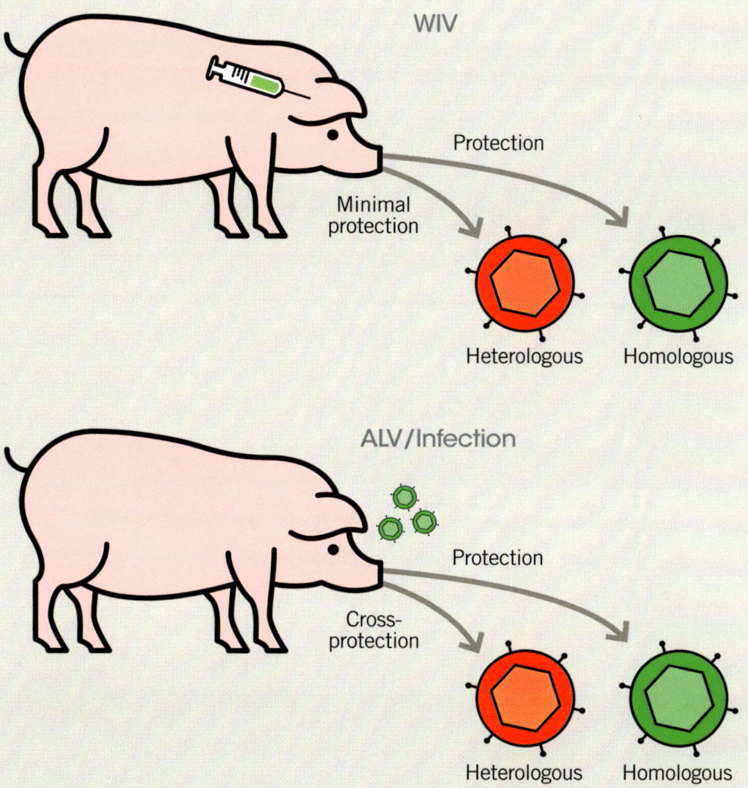

**Figure 18.** Excretion profiles in infected piglets and comparison of groups.
Average population profiles of viral excretion in piglets in direct and indirect contact with (a) MDA$^+$ and (b) MDA$^-$; (c) distribution of peak viral excretion by piglets in direct and indirect contact with MDA$_H^+$ (high), MDA$_L^+$ (low) and MDA$^-$ (Cador et al., 2016).

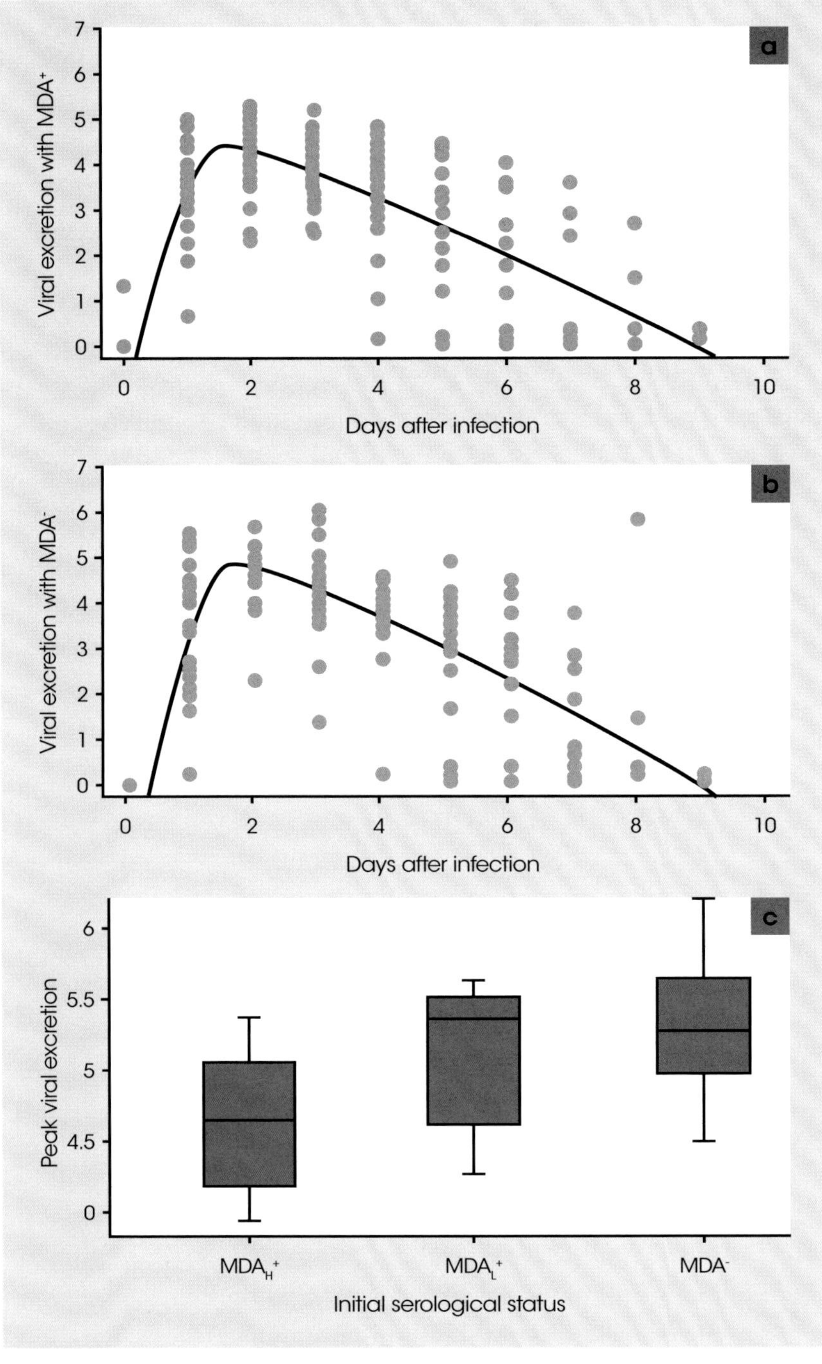

**Figure 19.** Serological profiles of porcine influenza type A in different piglet groups. Serological profiles (ELISA) in piglets with: high levels of maternal antibody that decrease continuously with no serological response to infection ($MDA_H^+$); low levels of maternal antibody that show a moderate serological response to infection ($MDA_L^+$); and no maternal antibodies, that show a significant serological response to infection ($MDA^-$) (Cador et al., 2016).

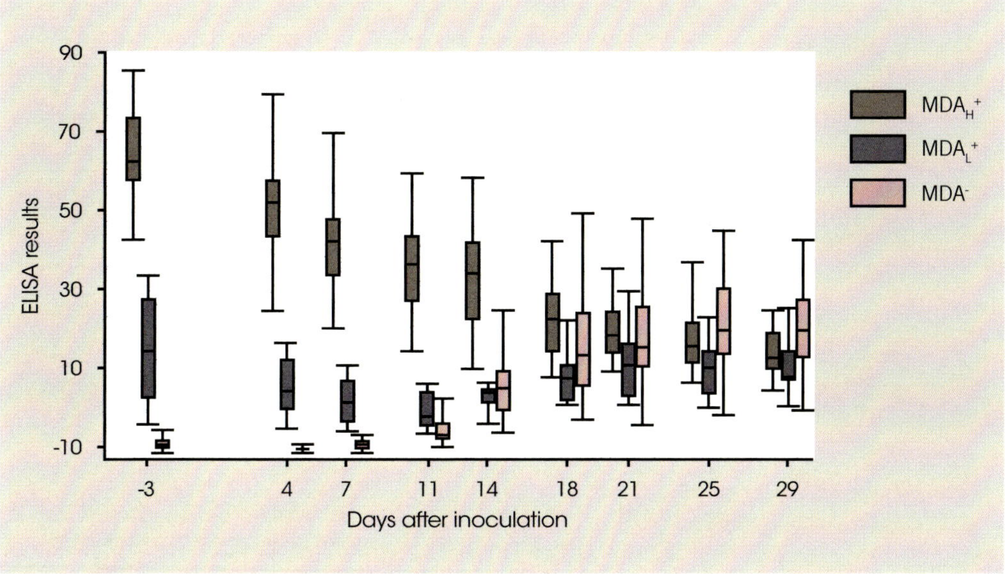

# 05

# PRACTICAL ASPECTS OF THE TRANSFER OF PASSIVE IMMUNITY TO THE PIGLET

# PRACTICAL ASPECTS OF THE TRANSFER OF PASSIVE IMMUNITY TO THE PIGLET

## MANAGEMENT OF COLOSTRUM CONSUMPTION

Colostrum is an essential source of nutrients for piglet survival during the neonatal period, providing humoral and cellular passive immunity as well as energy. As discussed at length in previous chapters, this passive immunity protects the piglet against pathogens until it is immunologically mature. The acquisition of passive immunity from colostrum occurs during the first 24–48 hours of life when the piglet can absorb the components of humoral and cellular immunity contained in the colostrum through the intestinal wall. The quality and quantity of colostrum administered to the piglet are therefore directly related to the passive immunity acquired, so factors that affect these parameters should be optimised.

### FACTORS RELATED TO QUALITY

Colostrum should contain components associated with humoral and cellular immunity to protect the piglet against the pathogens it may encounter during the neonatal period. This can be achieved if the sow has been exposed to these pathogens or vaccinated against them during gestation. Within the framework of the preventive medicine programme for the entire pig herd, specific strategies for gestating sows should be reviewed in depth. These programmes were presented in the previous chapter, and related to the main pathogens affecting pigs.

> Efforts should be focused on ensuring that gilts acquire enough humoral and cellular immunity for their colostrum to be as rich as possible, otherwise the piglets will be very susceptible to infectious diseases throughout the growing period.

## FACTORS RELATED TO QUANTITY

As discussed in depth in Chapter 3, piglets should ingest sufficient colostrum, estimated at approximately 250 g/piglet. Moreover, this colostrum should be sourced from the piglet's own mother to guarantee that the piglet acquires appropriate humoral and cellular immunity. Prolificacy has increased significantly on modern breeding farms due to intense genetic selection for this characteristic, and it is now very common to find farms with average prolificacy of over 15 piglets/sow (Fig. 1). This means that the sow needs to produce at least 3750 grams of colostrum to ensure that all her piglets can consume enough. The sow should be in good body condition to produce this amount of colostrum as colostrum production decreases when sows are excessively thin or fat. Finally, piglet management during the colostrum ingestion phase is extremely important to the acquisition of passive immunity.

The following conditions should be met for the piglet to be able to ingest sufficient colostrum:

- Sows should enter their farrowing accommodation 1 week before the anticipated farrowing date, to get used to the new environment to prevent stress during farrowing.
- It is advisable to feed a specific diet during the last week of gestation.
- Sow accommodation should be clean, disinfected and fully suitable for farrowing (Fig. 2).
- Piglets should be kept warm and dried as soon as possible, so drying materials should be at hand in the farrowing accommodation.
- Management by the staff attending farrowing is very important: staff should dry the piglets, guide them to the teats and assist in the birth if necessary.

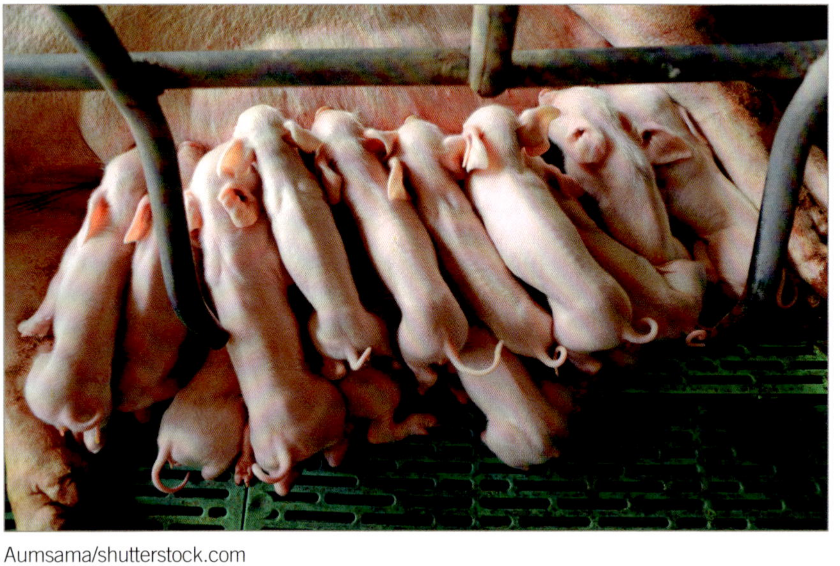

Aumsama/shutterstock.com

**Figure 1.** Hyperprolific sow.

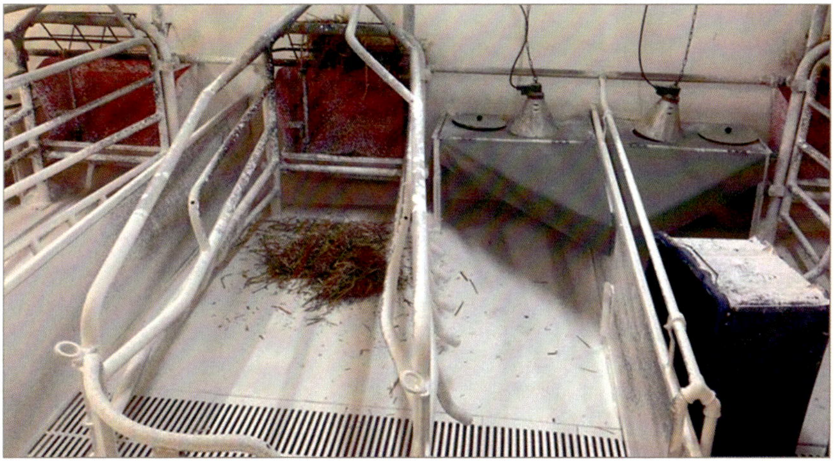

**Figure 2.** Suitable farrowing facilities.

- Every farm should implement a strategy to ensure that all piglets consume sufficient colostrum. Fig. 3 shows two sensible methods of achieving this objective. These methods can differ from farm to farm, but monitoring is essential to ensure that they are carried out correctly. It is also essential to allow piglets to remain with their mothers for at least 24 hours after birth.

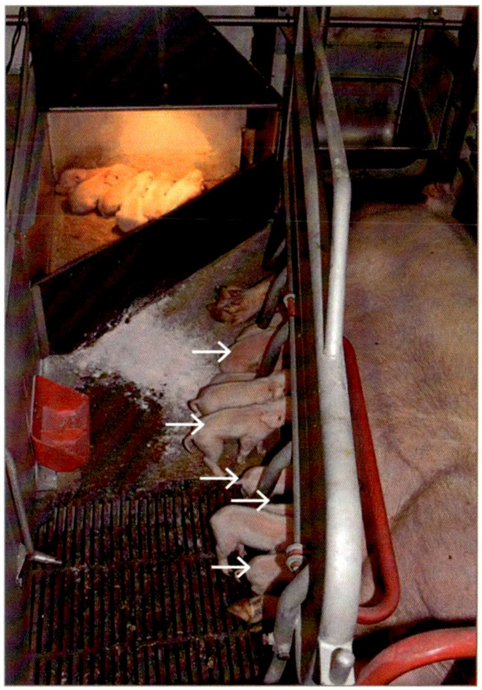

**Figure 3.** System to control colostrum consumption. First method: the biggest piglets are allowed access to their mother for 15 minutes/hour, while the 10 smallest piglets should remain with their mother all the time. Second method: the 5 smallest piglets are selected (arrows) and these should always remain with their mother. The biggest piglets are divided into 2 groups that are changed over every hour for the first 24 hours.

## MEASURING THE TRANSFER OF PASSIVE IMMUNITY

As mentioned previously, monitoring the ingestion of passive immunity is essential to optimise preventive medicine strategies in pigs. The techniques that can be applied in practice are described below, omitting any that are of academic relevance only. First, piglets can be weighed at birth and 24 hours after birth. Any weight gain is obviously due to colostrum consumption in the first day of life. There is even a prediction equation that relates the colostrum consumed to the weight gain. This technique is quite precise but is too laborious if there are many newborn piglets to be measured.

Another way of evaluating colostrum ingestion is to measure total serum IgG levels in the piglets at 24 hours old. As discussed previously, piglets are born agammaglobulinaemic and the level of IgG in the serum is directly related to the ingestion of colostrum. There is a technique that measures total IgG in pig serum, but it is not routinely performed by diagnostic laboratories so it is not directly accessible to farmers. One technique that has recently started to be used to evaluate colostrum intake by piglets is to determine the immunocrit. This method enables the amount of protein in the serum to be calculated by chemically precipitating the protein and calculating the proportion of precipitate to non-precipitate serum protein. As mentioned in previous chapters, most of the proteins in the piglet's blood in the first hours of life are immunoglobulins derived from the colostrum, especially IgG. Therefore, this method can be used after the piglet has ingested colostrum, as an indirect measurement of the colostrum immunoglobulins transferred from the mother to the piglet. There is an excellent correlation between immunocrit and plasma IgG levels in newborn piglets (Fig. 4).

Immunocrit can be used to indicate the level of passive immunity acquired by the piglet.

Not surprisingly, immunocrit values are related to stomach contents in newborn piglets, with low immunocrit levels linked to poor survival in the neonatal period, especially in piglets with low birth weights (Fig. 5). This method has been used experimentally to measure the transfer of passive immunity in piglets, but very few studies have been carried out on farm, so more trials are needed under real production conditions to evaluate the usefulness of this technique.

**Figure 4.** Relationship between immunocrit and IgG concentration in colostrum. Significant association ($p < 0.05$) and very high correlation can be seen between the two parameters ($r = 0.89$) which indicates that immunocrit is a suitable parameter to estimate the IgG concentration in the colostrum quite precisely (coefficient of determination of 78 %) (Vallet et al., 2017).

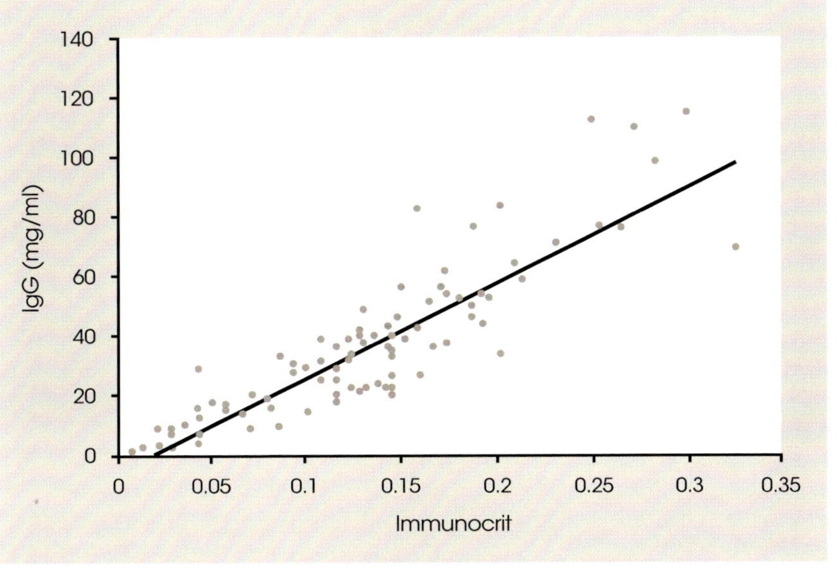


**Figure 5.** Relationship between immunocrit and preweaning mortality (Vallet et al., 2013).

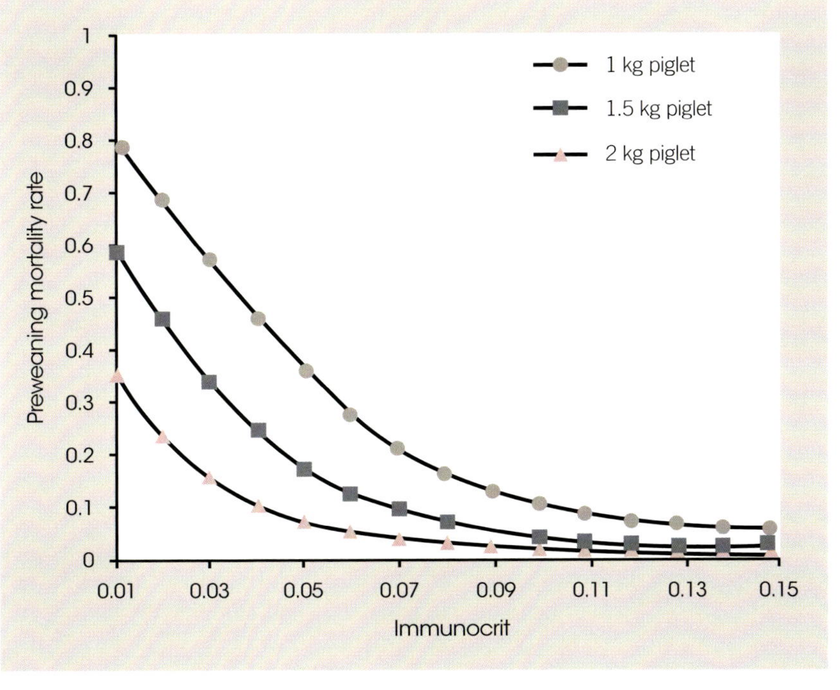

# REFERENCES

# REFERENCES


Adkins B, Leclerc C, Marshall-Clarke S. Neonatal adaptive immunity comes of age. *Nat Rev Immunol.* 2004; 4:553–564.

Adler B, Bulach D, Chung J et al. Candidate vaccine antigens and genes in *Pasteurella multocida. J Biotechnol.* 1999; 73:83–90.

Bandrick M, Pieters M, Pijoan C et al. Passive transfer of maternal *Mycoplasma hyopneumoniae*-specific cellular immunity to piglets. *Clin Vaccine Immunol.* 2008; 15:540–543.

Bandrick M, Theis K, Molitor TW. Maternal immunity enhances *Mycoplasma hyopneumoniae* vaccination induced cell-mediated immune responses in piglets. *BMC Vet Res.* 2014; 10:124.

Bandrick M, Ariza-Nieto C, Baidoo SK et al. Colostral antibody-mediated and cell-mediated immunity contributes to innate and antigen-specific immunity in piglets. *Dev Comp Immunol.* 2014; 43:114–120.

Barrios C, Brawand P, Berney M et al. Neonatal and early life immune responses to various forms of vaccine antigens qualitatively differ from adult responses: predominance of a Th2-biased pattern which persists after adult boosting. *Eur J Immunol.* 1996; 26:1489–1496.

Bazin H. A brief history of the prevention of infectious diseases by immunisations. *Comp Immun Microbiol Infect Dis.* 2003; 26:293–308.

Bertschinger HU, Fairbrother JM. *Escherichia coli* infections. In: Straw BE, D'Allaire S, Mengeling WL, Taylor D (Eds.), Diseases of Swine. Iowa State University Press, Ames, IA. 1999; 431–468.

Besser TE, Gay CC, McGuire TC et al. Passive immunity to bovine rotavirus infection associated with transfer of serum antibody into the intestinal lumen. *J Virol.* 1988; 62: 2238—2242.

Bossé JT, Janson H, Sheehan BJ et al. *Actinobacillus pleuropneumoniae*: pathobiology and pathogenesis of infection. *Microbes Infect.* 2002; 4:225–235.

Bourne FJ, Curtis J. The transfer of immunoglobins IgG, IgA and IgM from serum to colostrum and milk in the sow. *Immunology.* 1973; 24:157–162.

Brar JS, Johnson DW, Muscoplat CC et al. Maternal immunity to infectious bovine rhinotracheitis and bovine viral diarrhea viruses: duration and effect on vaccination in young calves. *Am J Vet Res.* 1978; 39:241–244.

Brockmeier SL, Register KB, Magyar T et al. Role of the dermonecrotic toxin of *Bordetella bronchiseptica* in pathogenesis of respiratory disease in swine. *Infect Immun.* 2002; 70:481–490.

Bruhns P, Iannascoli B, England P et al. Specificity and affinity of human Fc gamma receptors and their polymorphic variants for human IgG subclasses. *Blood.* 2009; 113:3716–3725.

Butler JE, Sun J, Weber P et al. Antibody repertoire development in fetal and newborn piglets. III. Colonization of the gastrointestinal tract selectively diversifies the preimmune repertoire in mucosal lymphoid tissues. *Immunology.* 2000; 100:119–130.

Butler JE, Weber P, Sinkora M et al. Antibody repertoire development in fetal and newborn piglets. VIII. Colonization is required for newborn piglets to make serum antibodies to T-dependent and type 2 T-independent antigens. *J Immunol.* 2002; 169: 6822–6830.

Butler JE, Francis D, Freeling J et al. Antibody repertoire development in fetal and newborn piglets. IX. Three pathogen-associated molecular patterns act synergistically to allow germfree piglets to respond to type 2 thymus-independent and thymus-dependent antigens. *J Immunol.* 2005; 175: 6772–6785.

Butler JE, Lager KM, Splichal I et al. The piglet as a model for B cell and immune system development. *Vet Immunol Immunopathol.* 2009; 128:147–170.

Cador C, Rose N, Willem L et al. Maternally Derived Immunity Extends Swine Influenza A Virus Persistence within Farrow-to-Finish Pig Farms: Insights from a Stochastic Event-Driven Metapopulation Model. *PLoS One.* 2016; 11:e0163672.

Cador C, Hervé S, Andraud M et al. Maternally-derived antibodies do not prevent transmission of swine influenza A virus between pigs. *Vet Res.* 2016; 47:86.

Cervenak J, Kacskovics I. The neonatal Fc receptor plays a crucial role in the metabolism of IgG in livestock animals. *Vet Immunol Immunopathol.* 2009; 128:171–177.

Chappuis G. Neonatal immunity and immunisation in early age: lessons from veterinary medicine. *Vaccine.* 1998; 16:1468–1472.

Chiers K, Van Overbeke I, De Laender P et al. Effects of endobronchial challenge with *Actinobacillus pleuropneumoniae* serotype 9 of pigs vaccinated with inactivated vaccines containing the Apx toxins. *Vet Quart.* 1998; 20:65–69.

De Jong MF. Progressive and nonprogressive atrophic rhinitis. In: Straw BE, D'Allaire S, Mengeling WL, Taylor D (Eds.), Diseases of Swine. Iowa State University Press, Ames, IA. 1999; 355–384.

Devillers N, Le Dividich J, Prunier A. Influence of colostrum intake on piglet survival and immunity. *Animal.* 2011; 5:1605–1612.

Donovan DC, Reber AJ, Gabbard JD et al. Effect of maternal cells transferred with colostrum on cellular responses to pathogen antigens in neonatal calves. *Am J Vet Res.* 2007; 68:778–782.

Ellis J, West K, Cortese V et al. Effect of maternal antibodies on induction and persistence of vaccine-induced immune responses against bovine viral diarrhea virus type II in young calves. *J Am Vet Med Assoc.* 2001; 219:351–356.

Endsley JJ, Roth JA, Ridpath J et al. Maternal antibody blocks humoral but not T cell responses to BVDV. *Biologicals.* 2003; 31:123–151.

Fablet C, Marois-Créhan C, Grasland B et al. Factors associated with herd-level PRRSV infection and age-time to seroconversion in farrow-to-finish herds. *Vet Microbiol.* 2016; 192:10–20.

Fablet C, Renson P, Eono F et al. Maternally-derived antibodies (MDAs) impair piglets' humoral and cellular immune responses to vaccination against porcine reproductive and respiratory syndrome (PRRS). *Vet Microbiol.* 2016; 192:175–180.

Fearon DT, Carroll MC. Regulation of B lymphocyte responses to foreign and self-antigens by the CD19/CD21 complex. *Annu Rev Immunol.* 2000; 18:393–422.

Ferrari CV, Sbardella PE, Bernardi ML et al. Effect of birth weight and colostrum intake on mortality and performance of piglets after cross-fostering in sows of different parities. *Prev Vet Med.* 2014; 114:259–266.

Firth MA, Shewen PE, Hodgins DC. Passive and active components of neonatal innate immune defenses. *Anim Health Res Rev.* 2005; 6:143–158.

Fraile L, Grau-Roma L, Sarasola P et al. Inactivated PCV2 one shot vaccine applied in 3-week-old piglets: improvement of production parameters and interaction with maternally derived immunity. *Vaccine.* 2012; 30:1986–1992.

Fraile L, Sibila M, Nofrarías M et al. Effect of sow and piglet porcine circovirus type 2 (PCV2) vaccination on piglet mortality, viraemia, antibody titre and production parameters. *Vet Microbiol.* 2012; 161:229–234.

Getahun A, Herman B. How antibodies act as natural adjuvants. *Immunol Lett.* 2006; 104:38–45.

Getahun A, Heyman B. Studies on the mechanism by which antigen-specific IgG suppresses primary antibody responses: evidence for epitope masking and decreased localization of antigen in the spleen. *Scand J Immunol.* 2009; 70:277–287.

Griebel PJ. Mucosal vaccination of the newborn: an unrealized opportunity. *Expert Rev Vaccines.* 2009; 8:1–3.

Haesebrouck F, Chiers K, Van Overbeke I et al. *Actinobacillus pleuropneumoniae* infections in pigs: the role of virulence factors in pathogenesis and protection. *Vet Microbiol.* 1997; 58:239–249.

Haesebrouck F, Pasmans F, Chiers K et al. Efficacy of vaccines against bacterial diseases in swine: what can we expect? *Vet Microbiol.* 2004; 100:255–268.

Heyman B, Nose M, Weigle WO. Carbohydrate chains on IgG2b: a requirement for efficient feedback immunosuppression. *J Immunol.* 1985; 134:4018–4023.

Heyman B, Pilstrom L, Shulman MJ. Complement activation is required for IgM-mediated enhancement of the antibody response. *J Exp Med.* 1988; 167:1999–2004.

Heyman B. Regulation of antibody responses via antibodies, complement, and Fc receptors. *Annu Rev Immunol.* 2000; 18:709–737.

Hjelm F, Carlsson F, Getahun A et al. Antibody-mediated regulation of the immune response. *Scand J Immunol.* 2006; 64:177–184.

Hodgins DC, Shewen PE. Vaccination of neonatal colostrum-deprived calves against *Pasteurella haemolytica* A1. *Can J Vet Res.* 2000; 64:3–8.

Hodgins DC, Shewen PE. Vaccination of neonates: problem and issues. *Vaccine.* 2012; 30:1541–1559.

Holmgren J, Czerkinsky C, Eriksson K et al. Mucosal immunisation and adjuvants: a brief overview of recent advances and challenges. *Vaccine.* 2003; 21:S2/89-S2/95.

Holt PG, Jones CA. The development of the immune system during pregnancy and early life. *Allergy.* 2000; 55:688–697.

Hurley WL, Theil PK. Perspectives on immunoglobulins in colostrum and milk. *Nutrients.* 2011; 3:442–474.

Ishikawa H, Kanamori Y, Hamada H et al. Development and function of organized gut-associated lymphoid tissues. J Mestecky, J Bienenstock, ME Lamm, L Mayer, JR McGhee, W Strober (Eds.), *Mucosal immunology* (3rd ed.). Elsevier, Amsterdam. 2005.

JONES C, POLLOCK L, BARNETT SM et al. The relationship between concentration of specific antibody at birth and subsequent response to primary immunization. *Vaccine.* 2014; 32:996–1000.

JUUL-MADSEN HR, JENSEN KH, NIELSEN J et al. Ontogeny and characterization of blood leukocyte subsets and serum proteins in piglets before and after weaning. *Vet Immunol Immunopathol.* 2010; 133:95–108.

KAAIJK P, LUYTJES W, ROTS NY. Vaccination against RSV: is maternal vaccination a good alternative to other approaches? *Hum Vaccin Immunother.* 2013; 9:1263–1267.

KARLSSON MC, GETAHUN A, HEYMAN B. FcgammaRIIB in IgG-mediated suppression of antibody responses: different impact in vivo and in vitro. *J Immunol.* 2001; 167:5558–5864.

KIM D, HUEY D, OGLESBEE M et al. Insights into the regulatory mechanism controlling the inhibition of vaccine-induced seroconversion by maternal antibodies. *Blood.* 2011; 117:6143–6151.

KLINKENBERG D, MOORMANN RJ, DE SMIT AJ et al. Influence of maternal antibodies on efficacy of a subunit vaccine: transmission of classical swine fever virus between pigs vaccinated at 2 weeks of age. *Vaccine.* 2002; 20:3005–3013.

KOVARIK J, SIEGRIST CA. Immunity in early life. *Immunol Today.* 1998; 19:150-152.

LE JAN, C. Cellular components of mammary secretions and neonatal immunity: a review. *Vet Res.* 1996; 27:403–417.

LECCE JG, MORGAN DO. Effect of dietary regimen on cessation of intestinal absorption of large molecules (closure) in the neonatal pig and lamb. *J Nutr.* 1962; 78:263–268.

LECLERC C. New approaches in vaccine development. *Comp Immun Microbiol Infect Dis.* 2003; 26:329–341.

LYUBCHENKO T, DAL PORTO J, CAMBIER JC et al. Coligation of the B cell receptor with complement receptor type 2 (CR2/CD21) using its natural ligand C3dg: activation without engagement of an inhibitory signaling pathway. *J Immunol.* 2005; 174:3264–3272.

MAES D, DELUYKER H, VERDONCK M et al. Effect of vaccination against *Mycoplasma hyopneumoniae* in herds with a continuous production system. *J Vet Med B.* 1998; 45:495–505.

MAES D, DELUYKER H, VERDONCK M et al. Effect of vaccination against *Mycoplasma hyopneumoniae* in pig herds with an all-in/all-out production system. *Vaccine.* 1999; 17: 1024–1034.

MARKOWSKA-DANIEL I, POMORSKA-MOL M, PEJSAK Z. The influence of age and maternal antibodies on the postvaccinal response against swine influenza viruses in pigs. *Vet Immunol Immunopathol.* 2011; 142:81–86.

MOREIN B, BLOMQVIST G, HU K. Immune responsiveness in the neonatal period. *J Comp Pathol.* 2007; 137:S27–S31.

MORRIS MC, SURENDRAN N. Neonatal Vaccination: Challenges and Intervention Strategies. *Neonatology.* 2016; 109:161–169.

MURPHY K, TRAVERS P, WALPORT M. *Janeway's immunobiology* (5th ed.) Garland Science, New York. 2001.

MURPHY K, TRAVERS P, WALPORT M. *Janeway's immunobiology* (6th ed.) Garland Science, New York. 2005.

MURPHY K, TRAVERS P, WALPORT M. *Janeway's immunobiology* (7th ed.) Garland Science, New York. 2008.

NECHVATALOVA K, KUDLACKOVA H, LEVA L et al. Transfer of humoral and cell-mediated immunity via colostrum in pigs. *Vet Immunol Immunopathol.* 2011; 142:95–100.

NGUYEN TV, YUAN L, AZEVEDO MSP et al. Transfer of maternal cytokines to suckling piglets: in vivo and in vitro models with implications for immunomodulation of neonatal immunity. *Vet Immunol Immunopathol.* 2007; 117:236–248.

NIEWIESK S. Maternal antibodies: clinical significance, mechanism of interference with immune responses, and possible vaccination strategies. *Front Immunol.* 2014; 16:446.

NIMMERJAHN F, RAVETCH JV. Fcgamma receptors as regulators of immune responses. *Nat Rev Immunol.* 2008; 8:34–47.

OBER RJ, RADU CG, GHETIE V et al. Differences in promiscuity for antibody-FcRn interactions across species: implications for therapeutic antibodies. *Int Immunol.* 2001; 13:1551–1591.

OSBURN B, STABENFELDT GH, ARDANS AA et al. Perinatal immunity in calves. *J Am Vet Med Assoc.* 1974; 164:295–298.

PARREÑO V, HODGINS DC, DE ARRIBA L et al. Serum and intestinal isotype antibody responses to Wa human rotavirus in gnotobiotic pigs are modulated by maternal antibodies. *J Gen Virol.* 1999; 80:1417–1428.

PLATT R, WIDEL PW, KESL LD et al. Comparison of the humoral and cellular immune responses to a pentavalent modified live virus vaccine in three age groups of calves with maternal antibodies, before and after BVDV type 2 challenge. *Vaccine.* 2009; 27:4508-4519.

POLEWICZ M, GRACIA A, GARLAPATI S et al. Novel vaccine formulations against pertussis offer earlier onset of immunity and provide protection in the presence of maternal antibodies. *Vaccine.* 2013; 31:3148–3155.

POMORSKA-MOL M, MARKOWSKA-DANIEL I. Interferon-gamma secretion and proliferative responses of peripheral blood mononuclear cells after vaccination of pigs against Aujeszky's disease in the presence of maternal immunity. *FEMS Immunol Med Microbiol.* 2010; 58:405–411.

POMORSKA-MOL M, MARKOWSKA-DANIEL I, PEJSAK Z. Evaluation of humoral and antigen-specific T-cell responses after vaccination of pigs against pseudorabies in the presence of maternal antibodies. *Vet Microbiol.* 2010; 144:450–454.

POMORSKA-MOL M, MARKOWSKA-DANIEL I, PEJSAK Z. Effect of age and maternally-derived antibody status on humoral and cellular immune responses to vaccination of pigs against *Erysipelothrix rhusiopathiae. Vet J.* 2012; 194:128–130.

QUESNEL H. Colostrum production by sows: variability of colostrum yield and immunoglobulin G concentrations. *Animal.* 2011; 5:1546–1553.

REBER AJ, LOCKWOOD A, HIPPEN AR et al. Colostrum induced phenotypic and trafficking changes in maternal mononuclear cells in a peripheral blood leukocyte model for study of leukocyte transfer to the neonatal calf. *Vet Immunol Immunopathol.* 2006; 109:139–150.

RODEWALD R, KRAEHENBUHL JP. Receptor-mediated transport of IgG. *J Cell Biol.* 1984; 99:159s–164s.

SABIN AB, ARECHIGA AF, DE CASTRO JF et al. Successful immunization of children with and without maternal antibody by aerosolized measles vaccine. II. Vaccine comparisons and evidence for multiple antibody response. *JAMA.* 1984; 251:2363–2371.

SAJI F, SAMEJIMA Y, KAMIURA S et al. Dynamics of immunoglobulins at the feto-maternal interface. *Rev Reprod.* 1999; 4:81–89.

SALMON H, BERRI M, GERDTS V et al. Humoral and cellular factors of maternal immunity in swine. *Dev Comp Immunol.* 2009; 33:384–393.

SEGALÉS J, URNIZA A, ALEGRE A et al. A genetically engineered chimeric vaccine against porcine circovirus type 2 (PCV2) improves clinical, pathological and virological outcomes in postweaning multisystemic wasting syndrome affected farms. *Vaccine.* 2009; 27:7313–7321.

SIBILA M, FRAILE L, TICÓ G et al. Humoral response and colostral antibody transfer following "one-dose" pre-mating vaccination of sows against porcine circovirus type-2. *Vet J.* 2013; 197:881–883.

SIEGRIST CA, CÓRDOVA M, BRANDT C et al. Determinants of infant responses to vaccines in presence of maternal antibodies. *Vaccine.* 1998; 16:1409–1414.

SIEGRIST CA, PLOTNICKY-GILQUIN H, CORDOVA M et al. Protective efficacy against respiratory syncytial virus following murine neonatal immunization with BBG2Na vaccine: influence of adjuvants and maternal antibodies. *J Infect Dis.* 1999; 179:1326–1333.

SIEGRIST CA. Neonatal and early life vaccinology. *Vaccine.* 2001; 19:3331–3346.

SIEGRIST CA. Mechanisms by which maternal antibodies influence infant vaccine responses: review of hypotheses and definition of main determinants. *Vaccine.* 2003; 21:3406–3412.

SIMISTER NE, MOSTOV KE. An Fc receptor structurally related to MHC class I antigens. *Nature.* 1989; 337:184–187.

SINCLAIR NR, LEES RK, ELLIOTT EV. Role of the Fc fragment in the regulation of the primary immune response. *Nature.* 1968; 220:1048–1049.

SINKORA M, SINKOROVA J, BUTLER JE. B cell development and VDJ rearrangement in the fetal pig. *Vet Immunol Immunopathol.* 2002; 87:341–346.

STIRLING CM, CHARLESTON B, TAKAMATSU H et al. Characterization of the porcine neonatal Fc receptor – potential use for trans-epithelial protein delivery. *Immunology.* 2005; 114:542–553.

STRAW BE, D'ALLAIRE S, MENGELING WL, TAYLOR DJ (Eds). *Diseases of Swine.* Ames, Iowa: Iowa State University Press. 1999.

TAYLOR D. Clostridial infections. In: Straw BE, D'Allaire S, Mengeling WL, Taylor D. (Eds.), *Diseases of Swine.* Iowa State University Press, Ames, IA. 1999; 395–412.

TAYLOR RB. Regulation of antibody responses by antibody towards the immunogen. *Immunol Today.* 1982; 3:47–51.

THACKER E, THACKER B, KUHN M et al. Evaluation of local and systemic immune responses induced by intramuscular injection of a *Mycoplasma hyopneumoniae* bacterin to pigs. *Am J Vet Res.* 2000; 61:1384–1389.

THEIL PK, LAURIDSEN C, QUESNEL H. Neonatal piglet survival: impact of sow nutrition around parturition on fetal glycogen deposition and production and composition of colostrum and transient milk. *Animal.* 2014; 8:1021–1030.

THEIL PK, FLUMMER C, HURLEY WL et al. Mechanistic model to predict colostrum intake based on deuterium oxide dilution technique data and impact of gestation and prefarrowing diets on piglet intake and sow yield of colostrum. *J Anim Sci.* 2014; 92:5507–5519.

THORNTON BP, VETVICKA V, ROSS GD. Function of C3 in a humoral response: iC3b/C3dg bound to an immune complex generated with natural antibody and a primary antigen promotes antigen uptake and the expression of co-stimulatory molecules by all B cells, but only stimulates immunoglobulin synthesis by antigen-specific B cells. *Clin Exp Immunol.* 1996; 104:531–537.

TIZARD IR. *Veterinary Immunology,* 8th edition. St Louis, Missouri: Saunders Elsevier. 2009.

TIZARD IR. *Veterinary Immunology,* 9th edition. St Louis, Missouri: Saunders Elsevier. 2013.

TUBOLY S, BERNÁTH S, GLÁVITS R et al. Intestinal absorption of colostral lymphoid cells in newborn piglets. *Vet Immunol Immunopathol.* 1988; 20:75–85.

TUBOLY S, BERNÁTH S, GLÁVITS R et al. Intestinal absorption of colostral lymphocytes in newborn lambs and their role in the development of immune status. *Acta Vet Hung.* 1995; 43:105–115.

VAN DEN BOSCH H, FREY, J. Interference of outer membrane protein PalA with protective immunity against *Actinobacillus pleuropneumoniae* infections in vaccinated pigs. *Vaccine.* 2003; 21:3601–3607.

VALLET JL, MILES JR, REMPEL LA. A simple novel measure of passive transfer of maternal immunoglobulin is predictive of preweaning mortality in piglets. *Vet J.* 2013; 195:91–97.

VALLET JL, MILES JR, REMPEL LA et al. Relationships between day one piglet serum immunoglobulin immunocrit and subsequent growth, puberty attainment, litter size, and lactation performance. *J Anim Sci.* 2015; 93:2722–2729.

VALLET JL, CALDERÓN-DÍAZ JA, STALDER KJ et al. Litter-of-origin trait effects on gilt development. *J Anim Sci.* 2016; 94:96–105.

VALLET JL, MILES JR. The effect of farrowing induction on colostrum and piglet serum immunocrits is dependent on parity. *J Anim Sci.* 2017; 95:688–696.

VINCENT AL, MA W, LAGER KM et al. Live attenuated influenza vaccine provides superior protection from heterologous infection in pigs with maternal antibodies without inducing vaccine-associated enhanced respiratory disease. *J Virol.* 2012; 86:10597–10605.

WARD LA, RICH ED, BESSER TE. Role of maternally derived circulating antibodies in protection of neonatal swine against porcine group A rotavirus. *J Infect Dis.* 1996; 174:276–282.

WATERS M, SAVOIE A, GRAMORY HS et al. Genotyping and phenotyping of β2-toxigenic *Clostridium perfringens* fecal isolates associated with gastrointestinal diseases in piglets. *J Clin Microbiol.* 2003; 41:3584–3591.

WEIBLEN R, WOODS GT, MANSFIELD ME et al. Comparative study of vaccines in preventing respiratory disease in beef calves after weaning. *Res Commun Chem Pathol Pharmacol.* 1982; 35:303–324.

WENG C, LIN W. Cell-mediated immune response in pig after *Mycoplasma hyopneumoniae* infection: effect of immunosuppression on pneumonia in pig induced by *M. hyopneumoniae. J Chin Soc Vet Sci.* 1988; 14:267–273.

WIERSMA EJ, COULIE PG, HERMAN B. Dual immunoregulatory effects of monoclonal IgG-antibodies: suppression and enhancement of the antibody response. *Scand J Immunol.* 1989; 29:439–448.

WOOD RL. Erysipelas. In: Straw BE, D'Allaire S, Mengeling WL, Taylor D (Eds.), *Diseases of Swine.* Iowa State University Press, Ames, IA. 1999; 419–430.

Wood N, Siegrist CA. Neonatal immunization: where do we stand? *Curr Opin Infect Dis.* 2011; 24:190–195.

Xue W, Ellis J, Mattick D et al. Immunogenicity of a modified-live virus against bovine viral diarrhea virus types 1 and 2, infectious bovine rhinotracheitis virus, bovine parainfluenza-3 virus, and bovine respiratory syncytial virus when administered intranasally in young calves. *Vaccine.* 2010; 14: 3784–3792.

Yoshida M, Masuda A, Kuo TT et al. IgG transport across mucosal barriers by neonatal Fc receptor for IgG and mucosal immunity. *Springer Semin Immunopathol.* 2006; 28:397–403.

Zhou X, Wang D, Xiong J et al. Protection of chickens, with or without maternal antibodies, against IBDV infection by a recombinant IBDV-VP2 protein. *Vaccine.* 2010; 28:3990–3996.